STRESS AND THE HEART
Storm in a Bottle

STRESS AND THE HEART
STORM IN A BOTTLE

Sander Orent, M.D.

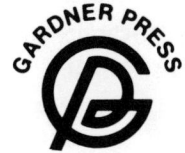

Gardner Press, Inc.
New York • London

Copyright © 1988 by Gardner Press, Inc.

All rights reserved.
No part of this book may be reproduced in any form,
by photostat, microform, retrieval system,
or any means now known, or later devised,
without prior written permission of the publisher.

Gardner Press, Inc., 19 Union Square West,
New York, NY 10003

Gardner Press Distributions
% M&B Fulfillment Services
540 Barnum Avenue
Bridgeport, CT 06608

Distributed to the trade by
Kampmann & Company, 9 East 40 Street
New York, NY 10016

All foreign orders except Canada and South America to:
Afterhurst Limited
Chancery House, 319 City Road
London N1, United Kingdom

Library of Congress Cataloging-in-Publication Data

Orent, Sander.
  Stress and the heart.

  Includes inces.
  1. Cardiovascular system—Diseases—Popular works.
2. Heart—Diseases—Psychosomatic aspects. 3. Stress
(Physiology) I. Title. [DNLM: 1. Heart Diseases—
etiology—popular works. 2. Stress, Psychological—
complications—popular works. WG 113 066s]
RC672.074 1988   616.1'2071   87-7540
ISBN 0-89876-139-5

Designed by Sidney Solomon

Printed in The United States of America

To Guenter Rose.

To the staff and my former colleagues at Franklin Memorial Hospital in Farmington, Maine, for their support and encouragement, and to my wife Deborah, for her fine illustrations, but mostly for her love.

CONTENTS

Preface

Introduction   1

1   Beginnings   7
2   Eye of the Storm: The Physiology of the Stress Response   15
3   The Ticking of the Clock: Type A Behavior and Coronary Heart Disease   25
4   Getting Ahead: Hurrying, Hostility, and Hyperreactivity   43
5   The Gathering Clouds: Tension, Hypertension, and Type A Behavior   63
6   The Storm Breaks: Coronary Heart Disease and Other Sequelae   87
7   Uncorking the Bottle: Does It Matter?   111
8   Umbrellas: Medicines, Movement, and Meditation   127
9   Rainbows   157

Glossary   171
Name Index   175
Subject Index   181

PREFACE

Stress is nothing new. It did not originate with human beings, nor will it pass with them. It is a ubiquitous fact of the biological world, an anvil upon which genetic characters are forged. It is that which pushes the living creature onward, away from placid existence. It is the causative force of biological change. Ultimately, the inability to adapt to stress is death, and successful adaptation is survival. Our animal kin are shaped by their stresses, not just in a genetic sense, but in their destinies as individuals as well. We, on the other hand, know stress for what it is. We are aware of the feeling stress awakens and hence are conscious of it. Stress begets creativity. It shapes our poetry, our music, our tears. We are unique in that by our awareness, by our will, we may channel stress—to some degree choose our response consciously, and hence affect our own destiny.

Stress is not bad or good; it is a fact of existence. This book is an attempt to examine this life-shaping force, this fact of life, and to place it in a perspective that will allow us to see how it molds our lives, and how we may consciously channel that process for our own evolutionary success.

INTRODUCTION

*I*t is often said that we live in stressful times. These are times marked by global political instability in the face of a looming shadow of nuclear holocaust, not to mention the more mundane pressures of employment insecurity, high-interest mortgages, rising food and gasoline prices, strikes, information overload, even dead car batteries and no aspirin in the medicine cabinet—the stresses of daily life. Are these afflictions of civilization, these by-products of technology, unique to our century, or even our decade?

We certainly are more aware than our ancestors, and far more concerned about life's stresses. Stress reduction, coping with stress, stress headaches, a stressful day at work, feeling "stressed out" all are common parlance involving a new use of a word that was once utilized primarily to describe the tensile strength of metal.

It is not clear that our stresses are any more profound today than in times of yore. If anything, the impact of physical stressors has been markedly lessened by technological comforts, from home heating oil to automotive transport. However, life circumstances appear more complex, interaction occurs with a wider variety of individuals, and information (and hence sources of worry) about the world in which we live is far more plentiful, also as a result of our access to technology. The jangling of a telephone can evoke much more than an auditory response to a ringing bell, simply because of who might be on the other end. The six o'clock news, on which we learn of a murder in an adjacent community, is far more effective in creating mass concern rapidly than was the over-the-fence information exchange of an earlier era.

INTRODUCTION

But despite this ubiquitous phenomenon of stress in our society, we live longer, healthier lives, on the whole, than at any time in history, and that trend is projected to continue until our maximum biological life span has been attained.[1] Even this barrier is being questioned and may prove to be not unsurmountable. We take vacations, have weekends off, and possess any number of sophisticated toys that distract us from the rigors of daily survival.

Thus it would appear that stress is not necessarily fatal, at least no more so than the infectious killers of the past we have so handily vanquished. This does not alter the fact, however, that stress can be detrimental to an organism: too much for too long can cause disease. Classical stress-related illnesses, such as irritable bowel syndrome and tension headaches, are not controversial as to their causality. Far more sinister are the implications that stress causes, or at least contributes to, heart disease and cancer, the first and second most important killers of modern Western men and women. This is an issue we examine in detail, for if stress indeed is a major causative factor in these two diseases, and we learn to deal with it effectively, of what then will we die?

Conversely, as we stated earlier, stress is a potent biological force without which there would be no evolutionary pressure, no change. This is intolerable in living systems, and is impossible in a nonconstant environment such as our planet (see discussion of homeostasis, Chapter 1). Stress can be a positive force capable of overcoming disease processes, a fact attested to by the potency of some of the "shock therapies" for certain diseases in common use at the beginning of this century, and which still have certain applications today.

Is this a paradox? Perhaps. But it is one that is resolvable, at least in part, by careful recognition of what we mean by stress and the situations in which it occurs. This will be the thrust of the first chapter.

There are many aspects of the stress response that involve most, if not all, body systems. This book is directed primarily to how the body prepares itself to deal *actively* with challenge, and the effects of this preparation on the heart and blood vessels, collectively termed the cardiovascular system. That this system is important and vulnerable is evidenced by the fact that cardiovascular disease, including coronary disease, hypertension, and its sequelae, is the

INTRODUCTION

primary killer of both men and women in the Western world.

In this book we are concerned with the cardiovascular stress responses of that rather complex ape, Homo sapiens. We shall be most interested in the behaviors of this organism as it copes with environmental realities quite divorced from its previous evolutionary experience, and how some of its responses to these new challenges might create disease. In Chapter 2 we detail the nature of the human cardiovascular stress response in such a manner as to permit a thorough grasp of physiologic principles by a nonscientist and to potentiate critical evaluations of the research work we present. We explore, in essence, the eye of the storm.

We then proceed to discuss specific behavioral patterns, termed "A" and "B." Chapters 3, 4, and 5 investigate respectively, the association of these behavior patterns with disease states, the mechanisms by which this might occur, and the potential ramifications for health. In Chapter 6 we synthesize this information into a model of stress-related cardiovascular disease, with some rather far-reaching implications. Chapter 7 is concerned with whether changing our responses to stress makes any difference in preventing disease.

In Chapters 8 and 9, we look at some ways to "keep the rain off," and more important, to keep the storm at bay. What this book will offer health-care providers is a thorough background in this most important area of psychosomatic medicine. This will enable them to educate and motivate their patients, and to derive and prescribe sound interventions, often without recourse to medication, and convince physicians, among others, of the validity of diagnosing and treating components of an illness that are not purely physical in etiology.

Before beginning, however, something should be said about the methods by which we reach our conclusions about this most controversial area of medical inquiry.

Science is an imperfect process. Experimental results are often perplexingly contradictory, which forces us to rethink and revise our ideas to accommodate data that do not fit neatly into our theories. The only other alternative is to ignore that which frustrates and confuses us, and pretend it never happened. The exception proves the rule, but invalidates the law. The value of conflicting medical results is that when an idea is challenged by data that do not fit, and experimental artifacts are ruled out as the cause, the idea must

INTRODUCTION

either be broadened in scope to enfold the new findings (hence enlarging its context) or it must be discarded and a new structure created that will fit the facts better. This is how scientific thought evolves—a process of survival of the truest and most consistent.

As we examine the issue of biological stress, we will look at what scientists are currently thinking; and this, by its nature, means there will be many theories, and a few gems of truth. Those rare gems will be polished and presented regally; however, much of what appears in these pages will be in the nature of theories, often with contradicting evidence that threatens to degrade laws to rules and facts to artifacts.

It would be gratifying to present a unified theory of disease with stress as a primary perpetrator. However, as we explore the relationship of stress and illness, we will see that the issue of causality is not nearly so simple. Despite Sontag's assertion that "the notion that a disease can be explained only by a variety of causes is precisely characteristic of thinking about diseases whose causation is not understood," we may find that causality is far more complex than we ever considered it to be. It is intellectually satisfying, though facile, to say that tuberculosis is caused by the tubercle bacillus. The disease tuberculosis is caused by the interaction of the bacillus with the host, and as such its ultimate expression is intimately connected to the host's nutritional status, the presence of other illnesses, previous exposures both individually and genetically, environmental circumstances (i.e., hygiene), and other factors, perhaps including "stress." To paraphrase Pasteur, "It is not so much the organism, but the *soil* that is important in creating disease." The state of that "soil" is complex and multifaceted. This does not mean that we are unable to draw valid and useful conclusions based on science's exploration of our subject. Indeed it is only by making the jump from the laboratory to the clinic on the basis, essentially, of inference that we will ever develop meaningful models of stress and disease.

Here, too, another warning is warranted: We must not be too quick to infer rules for humans on the basis of animal work, or rules for the many on the basis of data from the few.

Additionally, it is tempting to popularize scientific data to make them relevant and appealing to the lay public, and hence occasionally to render sensational conclusions that are not warranted. For in-

INTRODUCTION

stance, as Sontag so eloquently remarked,[2] "The hypothesis that distress can affect immunological responsiveness (and, in some circumstances, lower immunity to disease) is hardly the same as—or constitutes evidence for—the view that emotions cause diseases, much less the belief that specific emotions can produce specific diseases." Such misconstruals can have serious consequences for patients and families, as we discuss in a subsequent chapter.

Science is imprecise, but it is trying to be otherwise. It is the most stalwart force against the unknown available to us, replacing superstition with knowledge and deities with explanations. Therefore, I will be as true as possible to its principles, and will attempt to maintain objectivity in presenting the many aspects of stress, some apparently quite contradictory. Some of the paradigms presented herein are syntheses of data and principles across disciplinary lines and hence are somewhat unique; some of these syntheses were necessary in order to encompass apparently paradoxic information without ignoring the paradoxes. Let us begin.

1
BEGINNINGS

The body's systems, like any type of machinery, have certain requirements with regard to optimal operating temperatures, pressures, fluid levels, pH, oxygen concentration, and fuel supplies. These tolerances are fairly narrow, and a relatively constant internal environment is necessary for proper organ function. The body must attempt to maintain such inner constancy in the face of whatever storms rage around it in order to keep its organs functioning properly, in much the same way that a factory must be kept warm, lighted, and well ventilated. This process, the maintenance of internal constancy, is known as homeostasis.

If atmospheric temperatures were always maintained at 75°F, our homes would have little need of thermostats. Likewise, if our bodies were suspended in an environment of constant temperature, fed a constant supply of nutrients in the proper concentration, and made no movements, the maintenance of homeostasis would be relatively easy. Clearly this is not the case. We survive unaided in temperatures from below freezing to 120°F, from 20,000 feet above sea level to 20 feet below, and we can exist without food or water for days. Yet our internal environment is kept constant. Our homeostatic mechanisms are capable of handling a relatively wide range of environmental extremes with no conscious assistance.

When these systems are stressed to the point of being unable to make the necessary adjustments, we are so informed, and may modify our behavior accordingly to remove ourselves from the stressful environment. For instance, if the outside temperature falls to the point where the body is losing heat faster than it produces it, our homeostatic mechanism for regulation (located in a portion of the brain called the hypothalmus) senses this, and sends out nervous impulses. These constrict the blood vessels in the skin to reduce heat loss (closing the windows) and shivering may occur, which produces heat (turning on the furnace). If the furnace, coupled with insulation (fat), cannot keep the body at a standard operating temperature (98.6°F), we become increasingly aware of our plight and put on more clothes or go where it is warmer. If we can do neither of these, the result wil be a decrease in body temperature (hypothermia), eventually followed by death. Organ systems do not function at low temperatures, and at some point tissue freezes. Any furnace worth its oil must be able to keep the water pipes in the house from freezing; if the furnace is unable to do so, it is inadequately designed, or poorly adapted to the climate in which it is used. Likewise, some organisms, perhaps due to their genetic makeup, are able to tolerate cold better than others—they are better adapted to cold climates. Adaptation, then, can be defined as the homeostatic mechanisms available to the organism to deal with a given environmental fact of life. An adaptation is rather specific, that is, it is meant to maintain homeostasis in a given environmental circumstance, (cold). Adaptability, on the other hand, might be defined as the ability of the body to maintain homeostasis despite a range of environmental extremes. A polar bear is well adapted to a cold climate primarily because of its insulation, a structural adaptation to cold. A coyote is an adaptable organism because its homeostatic mechanisms allow it to survive in a wide range of environments. Humanity has been able to tolerate environmental extremes beyond its genetic or structural capabilities by adapting behaviorally (putting on a coat or building an igloo). Note that if an organism has no evolutionary experience with an environment, it is unlikely that it will possess adaptive mechanisms to cope with that environment. A tropical fish thrown upon an ice floe in the Arctic will freeze rather rapidly because neither it nor its evolutionary ancestors have had any experience with this particular environmental extreme.

An adaptation, then, is an organic structure, mechanism, or behavior specifically suited to cope with a given environmental circumstance. Adaptability is a statement of the flexibility of the organism. It refers to the capacity for adaptation; that is, the potential. An organism never really "knows" how adaptable it is until faced with a environmental challenge or "stressor". (We shall return to this word shortly.) The organism's potential adaptation will actualize only when it is confronted with the need for adaptation. According to evolutionary theory, it is theoretically possible for our tropical fish ultimately to adapt to the ice floe if suceeding generations of fish are gradually exposed to colder and colder climates, with the process of natural selection acting to bestow an advantage on those organisms which, by chance mutation, are better equipped to cope with the increasingly cold environment.

Adaptation, however, can occur in the individual as well, if it is "adaptable" enough successfully to meet its environmental challenge. Witness two marathon runners training for a high-altitude marathon. The first athlete has exercised in the mountains, at 8000–10,000 feet; the other has trained at sea level. If the race is run in the mountains, our altitude-adapted athlete will fare far better than the flat lander, who will probably lie gasping on the trail after the first few miles. The athletes are equally adaptable, but the first, by exposing himself to the environmental stress gradually and progressively, has allowed himself to adapt, whereas the second, with no personal experience with the stress, is unsuccessful in maintaining homeostasis.

Now let us coalesce our concepts of homeostasis and adaptation and define the word "stress" in biologic terms. Because we do not live in a world of constants, our homeostatic mechanisms are constantly called upon to make minute adjustments to our heart rate, breathing, fuel supply, blood pressure, etc. A stressor, in its broadest sense, can be looked at as any perturbation in the environment that requires homeostatic mechanisms to adjust. In our cold weather example, the decreased temperature is the stressor and the homeostatic mechanism (either behavioral or mechanical adjustment) is the organism's adaptation to it.

It becomes fairly obvious that virtually any change in the external environment that is brought to the attention of the organism's sensors, either conscious or unconscious, which then stimulate a response from the organism, could be termed a stressor. This definition, however, is too broad to be of much practical utility. Rather, we will consider a stressor to be any event that taxes the homeostatic mechanisms beyond their normal tolerance, and hence triggers additional physiologic response.

Notice that up until this point we have been using the words stress and stressor interchangeably. It is time to be more concise.

Stress has been variously defined as an event, a subjective sensation, a feeling, and as a response of the organism to an event. For clarity, let us assign stressful events in the environment the term "stressor," and the multiple responses of the organism to that stressor the term "stress response."

The details of this response, which include hormonal secretion by a number of glands and the activation of certain components of the central nervous system, are discussed in Chapter 2. The response seems designed to amplify homeostatic mechanisms in the face of a challenge by a stressor. Understanding the response and its activation is the key to understanding stress-related disease.

The generic term stress can be used to describe the phenomenon of stressor/organism interaction in a general sense: that is, when we speak of stress per se we mean a situation in which a stressor has induced a stress response.

Now what may tax one organism's homeostatic mechanism, and therefore be stressful to it, by our new definition may have no effect on another; for example, a naked man and a polar bear at the north pole. The naked man is very stressed whereas the polar bear is quite comfortable. Our polar bear, however, would be quite discomfited on a Florida beach—an unstressful circumstance for most of us. Stress, then, must be looked at in the context of the organism subjected to it. This is not only true between species, but for individuals within species as well (our two athletes in the high-altitude marathon). This leads us to our first rule:

Rule 1: "Stress is relative."

The adaptability of a given organism will in large part dictate how it "perceives" a stressor. Again this must be viewed in context. A coyote is an animal suited to a wide range of environmental extremes—it is an adaptable creature and will find a wider range of environments less stressful than would a tropical fish.

The organism's capacity for handling stress is a function of (1) the nature of the stress; (2) its past experience with the stress, both genetically (its evolutionary history) and within its lifetime; and (3) its adaptability if the stressor is a novel one with which it has had no experience.

Cold weather, as we have seen, is not a stressor for a polar bear. The organism is adapted to cold primarily as a result of its genetic constitution, which gives it its fur and its cold weather metabolism. Although we cannot say for certain, we infer from this that the polar bear evolved in a cold climate, and classic evolutionary theory would say that over millions of years, natural selection of animals that had the capability of existing in colder climates resulted in the characteristics of the polar bear as we know it. Evolutionary experience molded the bear's physical character and homeostatic mechanisms. The bear is historically adapted to cold. Now our bear is captured by a biologist for the Miami Zoo and transplanted to Florida, an event certainly beyond its evolutionary and personal experience. The survival of the bear in Florida will depend upon how effectively the zoo can provide a cold environment and whether the bear's homeostatic mechanisms can successfully adapt to heat.

Rule 2: Successful adaptation is a "cure" for stress.

If the bear is only partially successful in adapting, it will exist in a state of chronic stress and ultimately will become ill. The mechanism by which this illness might occur is the topic of subsequent chapters. Let us not, however, despair for the polar bear; like most mammals, it is fairly adaptable and chances are will do just fine in Florida—and may even grow to enjoy it.

As in most scientific inquiry, we cannot leave things relatively uncomplicated and speak of "stress" or "stressors" per se. Rather, it is useful, and probably necessary, to consider three distinct varieties of stressors.

A stressor that occurs once—that impacts the organism for a brief period and disappears—results in an *acute stress*. The body has had no experience with this stress, and successful coping will result only if the body's endogenous homeostatic mechanisms, which are already in place, are capable of meeting and overcoming the stressor so that internal constancy is not interrupted. Various components of the stress response seemed designed to aid this process. Traumatic injury is an example of an acute stress. Depending upon the severity of the injury sustained, homeostatic mechanisms will be taxed to the utmost. If they are successful in maintaining internal constancy within the parameters necessary to sustain life, the organism will survive and ultimately heal. If they are not, death will result. Aside from the severity of the injury, the only variable here is the state of the health of the organism prior to the incident. Other examples of acute stress are near-drowning, severe weather changes of short duration, or an acute infectious process, (such as pneumonia or the common cold). In the last case, the state of health of the organism is the major variable, because the immune system that fights off the infection seems intimately related to it.

A second broad category of stress is *chronic intermittent stress*. This results from a stressor that affects the organism acutely and repeatedly for discrete periods of time. It is not present constantly. An example of a chronic intermittent stress might be a loud noise that's repeated for five minutes every hour, such as a foghorn or jet planes at an airport. Chronic intermittent stress might also result from repeatedly performing a difficult task or repeated exposure to a stressful environment. Use of alcohol in large intermittent doses (binges) or cigarette smoking are also examples of chronic, intermittent stress. The effect of these agents will be primarily present when they are ingested. Such stressors are lessened in their impact by two phenomena. The first is adaptation—homeostatic mechanisms ''learn to live'' with chronic stress within the limits of their genetic competence. The second mechanism is anticipation of the stress and initiation of appropriate countermeasures. This might be termed learning. For instance, if one moved into a home next to an airport, the first night would be rather challenging to one's homeostatic mechanisms each time a jet took off or landed. Probably one's heart would race, blood pressure would increase, and eardrums would protest. In time one would learn the cues that would forewarn of a flyover, and the cardiovascular system would take it all in stride, one's hands would cover one's ears for the necessary interval, and life would go on as usual. One has ''learned'' and adapted. As we shall see, learning is a most important mechanism for adaptation to stress.

The third type of stress is *chronic persistent stress*. This transpires essentially without respite. Such a situation is most trying to an organism, and failure to adapt will result in the breakdown of homeostasis, the chronic activation of the stress response, and illness. Adaptation is the only cure, and if that is successful, the situation no longer will be stressful. Partial adaptation will delay, but not prevent, the ultimate sequelae of homeostatic failure.

An example of chronic persistent stress might be an environmental pollutant that is toxic to an organism. These are obviously increasingly ubiquitous in our environment, and hence increasingly inescapable. Another example might be a chronic infection such as tuberculosis. Adaptation to these chronic persistent stressors would require, in the case of pollutants, a metabolic pathway capable of degrading the substance to harmless cogeners. Infection would need the successful repulsion of the invader by the host, or, more rarely, the development of a symbiotic, relationship between the two.

Interestingly, most chronic persistent stressors are not physical but are, at least in humans, "psychological." By this we mean that the environmental circumstances that are not inherently physically dangerous are perceived as dangerous by the organism. The paper tiger of a lawsuit stresses homeostatic mechanisms just as surely (albeit in a different fashion) as a flesh-and-blood tiger. Job stressors, financial tribulations, and difficult interpersonal interactions all qualify as chronic persistent stressors.

If an organism perceives an event as threatening, it becomes so, and it appears to be that perception that elicits a stress response. We will discuss much experimental animal work and also studies on humans that document this point. Obviously this stress is under our potential control, and if perception evokes response, then perhaps perceptual change can result in adaptation—that is, if we do not perceive an event as stressful psychologically, our bodies will not perceive it as stressful physically. It is on this premise that much of the latter portion of this book is based.

Now we must examine just what constitutes the stress response and how such responses stave off or create illness, depending upon how successful they are in aiding adaptation. We undertake this task in Chapter 2. If you feel you have a thorough grasp of the physiology of the stress response, you may wish to skip to Chapter 3.

REFERENCES

Walford, Roy. *Maximum Life Span* New York: W. W. Norton, 1983.
Sontag, Susan. *Illness as Metaphor,* New York: Vintage Books, 1977.

2

EYE OF THE STORM: THE PHYSIOLOGY OF THE STRESS RESPONSE

The human (and indeed the mammalian) response to an acute or chronic intermittent stressor is rather stereotypic, but quite functional in a variety of challenge or threat situations. It is an "enabling" event that prepares the organism for episodic bursts of motor activity that are far more intense than normal daily behaviors. These activities are escape, or defensive or offensive behaviors for the purpose of avoiding a predator, procuring food, or defending territory, and they divert most or all body functions to this end.

Such a response evolved to cope more effectively with physical challenge or threat, and so has been termed "fight or flight." The effectiveness of the fight-or-flight phenomenon in enhancing physical abilities is described in such anecdotes as the mother who lifts a car from her child or the fighting prowess of a cornered animal. Somehow this stress response is capable of enhancing performance when triggered by fear or anger. Let us see how this might be so.

First described by physiologist Walter Cannon,[1] the response stems from the brain and a small gland that sits on top of each kidney, called the adrenal. A hormone called epinephrine, popularly known as adrenalin, and a neurotransmitter of similar structure called norepinephrine appear to be the active agents responsible for altering the body's physiology in ways we will describe.

Let us first differentiate a hormone from a neurotransmitter. A hormone is a chemical substance secreted by a gland, which is an organ that manufactures that substance. The chemical is secreted directly into the bloodstream, where it circulates throughout the body and attaches to tissues that possess a receptor for it, much as a key fits in a lock. As not all cells possess receptors for all hormones, the substances are somewhat specific in their actions. Once the receptor is engaged, a chemical change takes place in the cell that produces the hormonal effect (see Figure 1). For instance, the

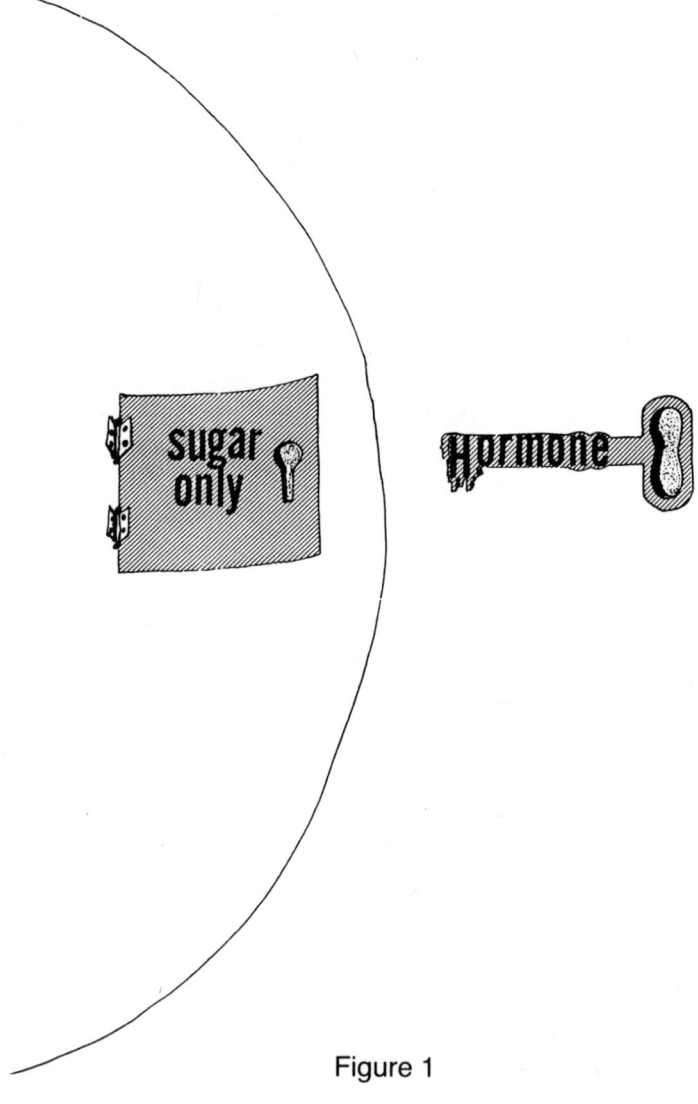

Figure 1

hormone insulin alters the cellular chemistry of some tissues to take up sugar as a fuel source. Without the hormone, the blood sugar levels build after a meal because the cells are incapable of utilizing this energy source. This is the diabetic state. Hormones act relatively slowly—over minutes—because they must circulate first.

Neurotransmitters are chemical substances secreted at the junction between one nerve fiber and another, or at the interface between a nerve and the structure or organ it innervates. It is released by an electrochemical phenomenon whose details are beyond the scope of our discussion, but the process is almost instantaneous. When the substance is released, it activates cells in a fashion similar to that of hormones, but only those cells actually supplied by the nerve that is discharging. Consequently, the response is much more specific and rapid (see Figure 2).

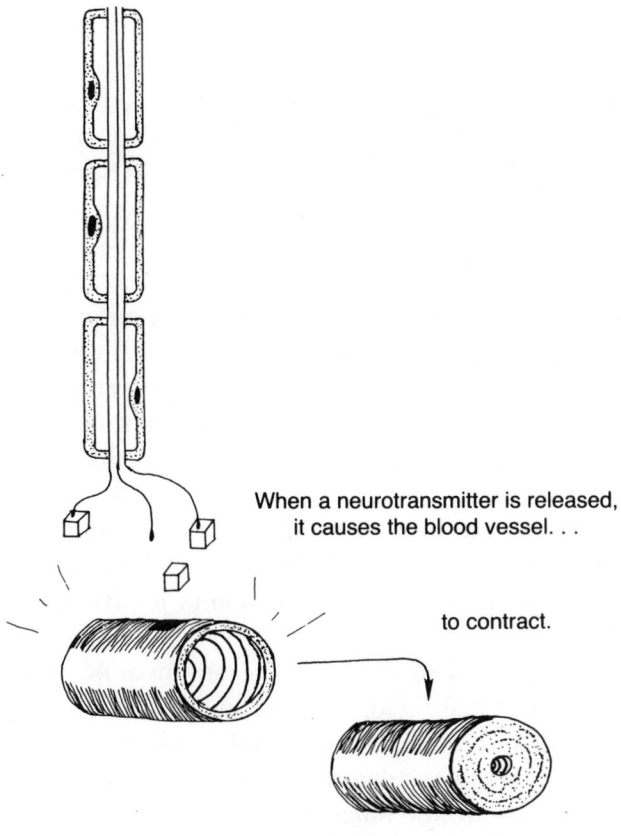

When a neurotransmitter is released, it causes the blood vessel... to contract.

Figure 2

Sometimes, as in the fight-or-flight response, hormone release is stimulated by nerve discharge, so that the instantaneous effect of the nervous activation is complemented by the slower, more general effect of the hormone release.

The fight-or-flight response, as we have mentioned, involves both hormones and nerves. There is a specific portion of the nervous system that has evolved solely and specifically to deal with the challenge of threat or injury, and is the central component of the stress response. This is called the sympathetic nervous system, and is not under voluntary control (note that certain "biofeedback" techniques, which are discussed in Chapter 8, can consciously alter some sympathetic functions). Another term for sympathetic is adrenergic. A counterpoint to the sympathetic system is the parasympathetic system, which calms the body down and deals with "vegetative" functions.

Let us envision the process as follows: We will create an analogy of the body as a factory whose output is movement and function. The factory must also be able to survive various disasters, such as floods and fires, and hence has various built-in safety mechanisms, such as drains and sprinklers. The factory should be able to change its output to meet demand, and have adequate storage capabilities for raw materials.

Our factory, as an assembly line of sorts, has a system of conveyor belts, both to supply materials and to remove wastes from manufacturing processes. This is the vascular system. The system has a good deal of shunting capability so that it can direct material and fuel supplies to areas most active at a given time. The arteries, or input pipes, are supplied with musculature that can vary the diameter of the pipes, and even shut off flow to certain regions altogether, on the basis of need. The central driving engine that moves all materials is the heart. There is no backup engine. The engine itself is well supplied with conduits for its own fuel consumption.

Energy is supplied in the form of carbohydrate and fat fuels; when the output of the factory is movement, these fuels are preferentially shunted to the pistons and pulleys (muscles). As in every fuel system, oxygen is needed for combustion, and is provided by a dual bellows system, the lungs. Oxygen is carried in the conduits in special tanks called red blood cells, where it is bound to a chemical called hemoglobin.

The factory is hard-wired rather extensively, which permits the factory executive to vary intake and output according to perceived external market demands. In addition, two automatic systems have been installed. The first, the parasympathetic, sees to the day-to-day operations such as fuel intake and storage (digestive processes) and baseline pump function, as well as "weekend" or resting energy distribution. It is basically a "low-gear system."

The second system is an emergency system that operates either when there is an extreme demand for movement output or when an internal disaster overwhelms the capabilities of the small local "fire extinguishers" situated throughout the plant (minor homeostatic adjustments). If, for instance, one of the conduits springs a leak that cannot be plugged locally, the system is activated. A characteristic of this sympathetic system is "mass discharge;" that is, when activated, most or all of its components are triggered simultaneously.

Let us look at the details of this emergency system. It is basically a "high gear" for the factory that is designed to produce maximum output in the shortest possible time, often under adverse conditions. As such, it must mobilize and appropriately distribute resources, maximize muscle output, and generate alertness on the part of all sensors. If the factory is attacked, it must repair the damage, plug the holes, and escape the damaging environment.

Despite the mass discharge activation characteristic of the sympathetic nervous system, there is some degree of differential wiring. Norepinephrine and epinephrine activate somewhat different receptors, and some receptors inhibit, whereas others excite, tissue function. For instance, some relax blood vessels and others contract them, so that sympathetic discharge will direct blood flow to certain areas and shut off others. This is not a yin/yang arrangement, in that sympathetic discharge strives to a common goal. Dilation in one tissue (i.e., an exercising muscle) is useful and vessel constriction to the skin is useful as well, to decrease bleeding in the case of laceration (see Figure 3). The same tissue does not have both constricting and dilating sympathetic receptors. Rather, the yin/yang is sympathetic/parasympathetic, with the two systems offsetting each other.

The sympathetic nervous system receptors are of two basic types—alpha and beta—and might be thought of as master switches.

EYE OF THE STORM

Norepinephrine, the neurotransmitter, primarily throws the alpha switch, and epinephrine the beta. (Note that this is not absolute; epinephrine triggers approximately 80 percent beta, 20 percent alpha-receptors) Alpha-receptors are concerned primarily with distribution, and so vary the diameter of the conduits. Most of the time, the consequence of alpha-receptor stimulation is to constrict the pipes, and hence decrease blood flow to a given region. These

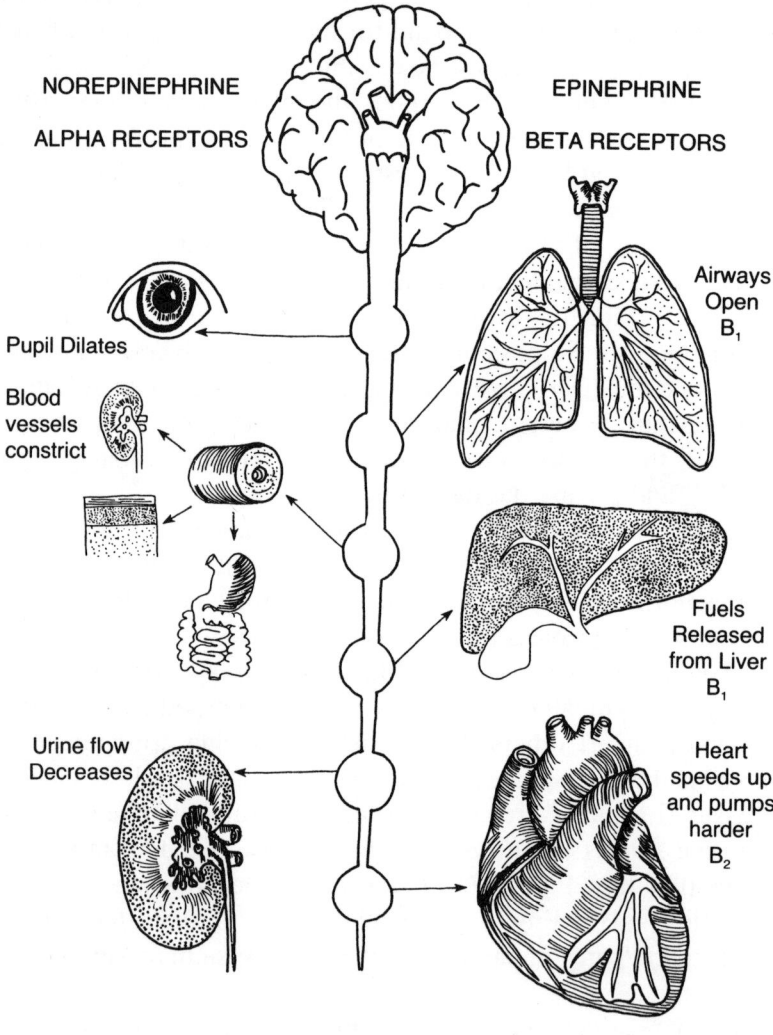

Figure 3

receptors are found in the skin and the gastrointestinal tract, as well as the kidney. Their stimulation can prevent blood loss in case of injury, and raise the pressure in the pipes elsewhere because of increased resistance to flow and the shunting of blood from these less immediately vital areas. Other alpha effects are to dilate the pupils, thus improving sensory intake, and to clamp closed urinary and intestinal sphincters to prevent accidental dumping of waste. In addition, the output of urine by the kidneys (filters) is decreased in an attempt to conserve inner fluid volume.

Beta receptors come in two categories: beta-1 and beta-2. Beta-1 switches primarily affect the pump, speeding its rate and force of contraction. Beta-2's activate fuel mobilization by mobilizing fat from storage depots and sugar from the liver, and dilate certain conduits, which increases fuel and oxygen input to the pump and musculature of the body factory. In addition, the bellows are stimulated to work faster, and oxygen conduits (airways) to open wide.

Some general sympathetic effects that are not clearly alpha or beta involve increased mental alertness, increased muscle strength, higher metabolic rate, and increased sweating (opening of the vents). Blood clots faster as a result of sympathetic nervous system activation as well.

There is no known natural mechanism for selectively turning on beta-1 versus beta-2 receptors, but this can be done artificially with certain drugs, as discussed in Chapter 8.

When the entire system is activated, we call this sympathomedullary arousal.

We alluded previously to executive decisions in factory output. The "executive" in the body to which we are referring, is, of course, the brain. Decisions with regard to sympathomedullary arousal are not truly conscious, but are more of the nature of reflex, triggered by input from sensory structures such as eyes, ears, or pain fibers. In fact, we cannot consciously command an "adrenalin rush," but only put ourselves in situations, such as sky diving, where activation of the sympathetic nervous system is likely to occur. When the response is not stimulated by fear, we tend to enjoy this alert, aroused state (adrenalin "high").

If pathology arises from repeated activation of this system, it may be due to the fact that humans become physiologically aroused by psychological or psychogenic challenge in the same stereotypic manner as if the challenge or threat were physical. We will spend much time investigating this premise.

There are a few other concepts of homeostasis and sympathetic nervous systems activation we need to address. The first involves the concept of the feedback loop. If output of a given material falls below the need for that material, our factory, to be efficient, would do well to have sensors on line that report this fact. Even more efficient would be the elimination of the chain of command, so that the defect did not have to be reported to a supervisor, etc., and orders relayed to increase production of the material. Rather, if the sensors could simply trigger a switch that would increase the supply of the materials directly from stores that would cease only when the sensors detected normal levels, the efficiency would be improved. For instance, if the blood sugar drops in the face of increased demand, body sensors can detect this and secrete substances that mobilize sugar from stores in the liver (see Figure 4). The analogy to a thermostat should be apparent. The feedback loop is a primary mechanism of homeostatic maintenance in the human body. Sensors exist for blood pressure, blood volume, various blood salts and

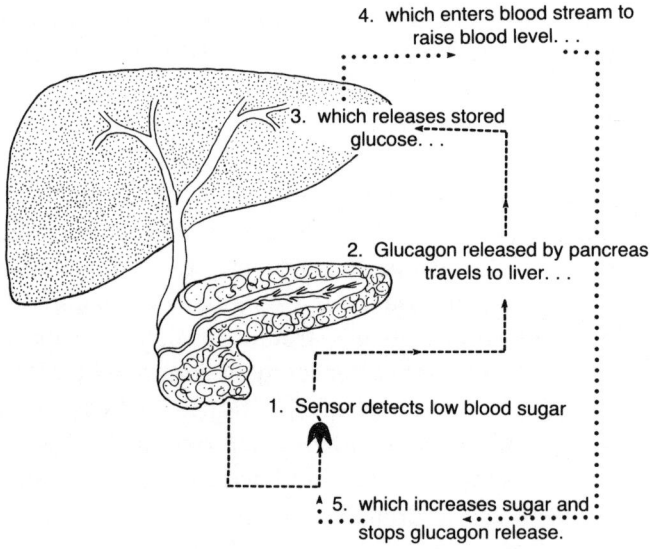

Figure 4

nutrients, muscle tone, hormone concentrations, and temperature, to name a few. When these sensors are not satisfied by a return to normal of the parameter they sense, the stress response may be activated. The mass discharge that ensues will in all likelihood enhance the normalization of that parameter, if it is an important body function. If sympathetic discharge is not stimulated by an internal emergency but by an external threat, it seems that the sensors are "reset" at higher levels by the sympathetic nervous system to compensate for the anticipated extreme demands on the organism (see Figures 5 and 6).

A second concept is that of prioritization. The body will preferentially maintain blood pressure at the expense of flow to nonvital organs, such as the gastrointestinal tract, if the volume of blood is depleted. Flow to vital organs such as the heart and lungs is maintained at virtually all cost. Blood salt concentrations give ground before total body fluid levels. Core temperature is prioritized over that of the skin. Sympathetic activation functions to ensure priorities by the location and nature of adrenergic receptors, which are designed to ensure these priorities.

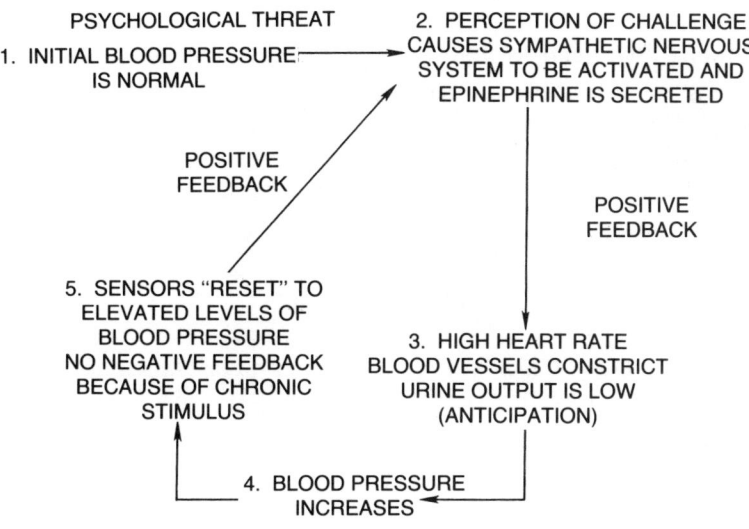

Figure 5

EYE OF THE STORM

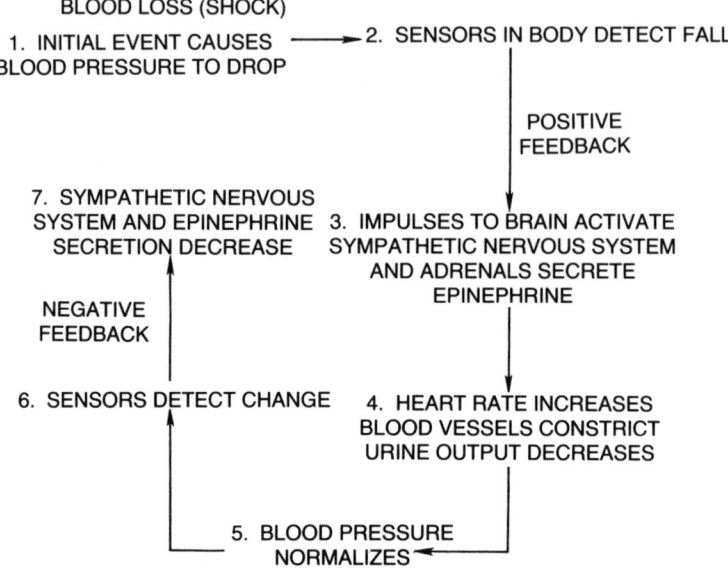

Figure 6.

Finally, we need to note the fact that sympathomedullary activation is not the only stress response available to the organism to cope with stressors. Chronic stress particularly can engage a different repetoire of hormones and neurotransmitters. However, in this book we focus on the impact of stress on the cardiovascular system. Thus let us meet our first patient, Mr. A.

REFERENCE

Cannon, W. B. *Bodily Changes in Pain, Hunger, Fear and Rage* (2nd ed.). New York: Appleton-Century, 1936.

3

THE TICKING OF THE CLOCK: TYPE A BEHAVIOR AND CORONARY HEART DISEASE

*M*r. A, a previously healthy 45-year-old business executive, finished dinner and was somewhat perturbed to notice a heavy, pressure-like sensation in his chest. Despite his self-assurance that it was his usual indigestion, it progressed to a viselike agony that numbed his left arm and made his jaw ache. He began to sweat profusely, became frightened, and drove himself to the local emergency room, where an electrocardiogram confirmed the diagnosis of acute myocardial infaction (a heart attack).

Evincing surprise upon learning the nature of his symptoms, Mr. A protested vigorously that he had never had a sick day in his life, did not smoke, played racquet ball twice a week, and had no family history of heart disease. His thorough (and expensive) physical done six months previously, which included an electrocardiogram, was completely normal, and so he could not understand how such a diagnosis was possible.

Classical medical doctrine, up until fairly recently, would have been hard-pressed to offer Mr. A an adequate explanation. He and his physician were correct in their assessment that he possessed few of the classic risk factors for the development of coronary atherosclerosis—the process of progressive occlusion of the feeder arteries to the heart muscle with calcium, cholesterol, and blood clots that ultimately results in a heart attack. Such risk factors—smoking,

25

hypertension (high blood pressure, not an excess of tension), a family history of heart disease, and elevated cholesterol content of the blood—are surely the most important predictors of the risk of myocardial infarction. Physical inactivity and corpulence have been implicated as well.

Mr. A, however, had none of the characteristics, except that he was unsure about his cholesterol. As he awaited his transfer from the emergency room to the coronary care unit, his pain somewhat eased by intravenous morphine, he began to think about all the jobs that would not be done during the two-week hospital stay the physician assured him he would be facing. He thought of the advertising deadline a week from Wednesday, the meeting scheduled for the following morning where his presence was indispensable, the new trainee who would surely be inadequate, and the reactions of his boss to the news of his incapacity. He glanced at his watch, and the date displayed thereon again evoked a vision of schedules and deadlines. An astute nurse, noting an increase in Mr. A's pulse as indicated on the monitor, gently suggested he try to relax.

Actually, this was not a new scenario for Mr. A. He had fantasized his incapacity many times in the past, a train of thought that generally made him more anxious to accomplish certain goals as rapidly as possible.

This also is not a new scenario for most health-care providers who deal with patients like Mr. A at some point during their illness, either during the acute hospitalization, or later for nutritional, psychological, or physical rehabilitation. Most of us recognize a certain behavioral constellation in these patients if not in ourselves.

Mr. A was displaying a style of relating to events and individuals in his environment that has been termed the Type A, or coronary-prone, behavior pattern. As early as 1868, it was noted that loud vocalizing and excessive work involvement predisposed to the development of coronary heart disease(CHD).[1] William Osler, who has been called the father of modern diagnostic medicine, noted in 1892 an association between hard-driving behavior and coronary heart disease.[2] In the 1930s, 1940s, and 1950s, a few similar observations appeared in the medical literature.[3-5]

Because of a failure to explain all, or even most, of coronary heart disease cases on the basis of the "classic" risk factors of smoking, hypertension, family history, and high serum cholesterol, these early observations were revived, and have been expanded and expounded upon quite intensely over the past three decades. This intensity is related to the dramatic increase in the frequency of this disease over the same time period to its position of prominence as the primary cause of death in the United States today.[6]

Observations of the behavior of patients at risk for, or possessing, a diagnosis of coronary heart disease (of which myocardial infarction and death are such grim end points) have coalesced into the concept of the Type A behavior pattern (TABP), typified by Mr. A. Dr. Ray Rosenman,[7] a contemporary researcher in the field whose work is among the most definitive, characterizes it thus:

> Individuals who are engaged in a relatively chronic struggle to do and achieve more in less and less time, often in competition with other people or opposing forces in the environment, exhibit the set of behaviors known as the Type A behavior pattern. The TABP includes such behavioral dispositions as ambitiousness, aggressiveness, competitiveness, and impatience; specific behaviors such as alertness, muscle tenseness, rapid and emphatic speech stylistics; and emotional reactions such as enhanced irritation and expressed signs of anger.

Other terms have been used to describe this mode of relating to the environment include hard-driving, time conscious, intense striver, pressured, excessively hostile, overachieving, and abrupt. The individual who is displaying Type A traits is likely to interrupt you before you have finished your sentence, glance frequently at his or her watch, fidget, and otherwise make you aware of the person's impatience and sense of urgency. Therapeutically we have all contacted such patients, but it is possible to be fairly precise about the nature of the pattern. The importance of this will be evident as we explore components of "A'ness" and attendant greater or lesser risk.

Two crucial points should be made here:

1. The TABP is exactly that—a pattern of behavior, not a personality characteristic. It refers to a mode of interaction with the environment that is evoked by events or circumstances that are perceived as challenging or threatening. As an evoked behavior, it is present episodically and circumstantially, and is not a fixed and invariable trait. This sounds suspiciously like the relationship of a stressor (perceived environmental challenge or threat) to a stress

response (the TABP). One might even speculate that this behavior pattern may have evolved as a method of procuring resources in a competitive world where food, mates, and shelter were limited in availability. Is this the link by which stress might contribute to the development of heart disease? We shall see presently.

2. Type A behavior is not an all-or-none phenomenon—that is, a given individual may display certain components of the behavior pattern (for instance, ambition) without excessive hostility or pressured speech. A particular pattern within the Type A framework may be quite consistent, and some researchers have proposed subclassifications such as A1 and A2, depending on the components present.[8] This, too, is not incompatible with the idea of Type A behavior as a stress response, for, as we have seen, stress responses are variable in their expression, between and within individuals.

The Type B behavior pattern has been defined as characterizing those individuals who do not display Type A behaviors.[7,9] This, of course, tells us what Type B is not, and succinct definitions are harder to come by, but essentially such an individual is more "laidback," rolls with the punches, and is more passive in any interactions with the world. Such individuals have been said not to be coronary-prone.

All of this seems to fit nicely into a fairly straightforward newly defined risk factor for coronary heart disease, the validity of which we can almost intuitively sense. It is the hard-driving, pressured soul whose excessive zeal finally results in a heart attack, and whose candle, having been burned at both ends, is extinguished prematurely. It is the sort of model relished by clinicians because it would seem to explain previously inexplicable phenomena (the occurrence of coronary heart disease in the absence of classical risk factors) and is associated with that "ah" of conceptual sensibility, the "of course" of understanding. But fortunately for the scientific process, it is the hobby of many scientists to subject new models to the target range of skeptical scrutiny; to shoot holes, as it were, in the soundest of theorems. The situation is indeed not so straightforward or the model as perfect as it first appears. Let us examine the evidence for the validity of the association between Type A behavior and coronary heart disease. Once this is established we can begin to look at casuality, but despite our clinical or intuitive judgments we must be sure such an association is real.

Our investigation must proceed in three stages: First, exactly what is the association between the TABP and coronary heart disease? With what frequency do they occur together? Do Type B individuals suffer from coronary heart disease? If so, do they do so less frequently than Type A's? Are there specific components of the Type A pattern that predict coronary heart disease better than others? Is there an association between the degree of Type A behavior and the severity of the disease?

Next, we must inquire as to what mechanisms such an association might occur (if it does). Is there a cause-and-effect relationship or merely an association between two conditions, both of which might be hereditarily linked? Is there a third variable common to both that might explain their association? If the TABP is indeed a form of stress response, is there an underlying and familiar physiologic process that might account for its seeming ability to "cause" heart disease?

Finally, assuming that a cause–effect interaction is found, does modification of one alter the severity or incidence of the other? Are there by implication interventions that might temper an (inappropriate) stress response and obviate its effects on its target organs (the heart and vasculature)? This, of course, is the key issue that might convince us and our clients that behavioral change could indeed prevent morbidity or an early demise from this disease.

Let us begin with a brief look at how the TABP and coronary heart disease are diagnosed and quantified. Type A behavior is assessed in two quite different (and not always concordant) fashions. The first, and simplest, technique is a self-administered questionnaire called the Jenkins Activity Survey.[10] This consists of a series of multiple-choice questions that are weighted by a point system that generates a score expressed as a percentage of Type A characteristics displayed by an individual. Questions deal with such subjects as the frequency with which one encounters deadlines in one's job, how much pressure such deadlines carry, and how many of these deadlines are self-imposed. Others explore one's own and one's spouse's perceptions of urgency and time pressure, feelings about being late or having to wait, how one spends one's time, and related issues.

The other most commonly used method of Type A diagnosis is

a more dynamic process entitled the Rosenman and Friedman Structured Interview.[8] As previously mentioned, the behavior pattern is an evoked one, and requires an appropriate challenge for its full expression. Generally these challenges are most effective when they confront an individual's sense of control,[11] present challenging or competitive tasks,[12-14] or threaten self-esteem.[12] The Structured Interview was designed to provide a relevant challenge in both its content and its pressured manner of administration. It is a one-on-one interaction with set content and manner of delivery, where responses are analyzed according to their content, style of speech, and nonverbal "body language" indices such as facial expression and use of the hands. The Structured Interview has been shown to be a more effective predictor of CHD incidence than the activity survey.[15] The ability to evoke Type A behavior consistently by challenge is most useful when we set about to study the consequences of this behavior in a laboratory setting, as we shall see. A number of other tests have been developed to attempt to quantitate the TABP, but in general have received somewhat less acceptance than those described.

It should be pointed out that the correlation between the Structured Interview and Activity Survey assessment of the TABP is moderate, which indicates that they are probably measuring somewhat different characteristics.[9-16-17] Therefore, it is necessary to view any study of this matter in the light of the assessment utilized. For instance, the Activity Survey was standardized to an employed, urban male norm; hence studies that examine a broader based population would be prone to certain inaccuracies on this basis. From a clinical perspective, the JAS is easier to administer, whereas accurate, reproducible analysis of the structured interview requires specific training available only at select medical centers.

There are many ways to diagnose coronary heart diease. The event of a myocardial infarction is generally considered diagnostic of coronary heart disease, except in those rare cases where the event is due to spasm of the coronary vessels, without associated atherosclerosis. The presence of a rather typical pain syndrome, known as angina pectoris, which is the pain of coronary insufficiency that occurs when demand of the heart for oxygen exceeds supply that is limited by narrowed vessels, is considered a manifestation of coronary heart disease. This syndrome is generally accompanied by characteristic changes on the electrocardiogram, the record of electrical potentials occurring in heart muscle, and can be provoked by an exercise tolerance test, where the electrocardiogram records responses during progressive treadmill exercise. The gold standard for the diagnosis of coronary heart disease is, however, the coronary angiogram, or arteriogram. In this test a radio-opaque dye that is visible on x-ray film is injected into the coronary arteries by means of a catheter threaded up an artery of the leg into the heart. A rapid progression of x-rays records the course of the dye through the vessels, and any areas of narrowing or occlusion due to atherosclerosis are evident. The extent of the narrowing can be quantified and the severity of coronary heart disease assessed.

Does Type A behavior predict coronary heart disease? Clear and repetitive research reported in the medical literature demonstrates a frequent and consistent association between these two phenomena. The fact that this is so lends validity to the premise, as the association is present across a variety of populations, in a variety of nations, and holds true for a variety of measures of both coronary heart disease and Type A behavior. The earliest studies retrospectively matched Type A characteristics with established cases of coronary disease, as manifested by either a history of myocardial infarction or the presence of angina. Many of these studies were European, and attempted to separate the various components of the behavior pattern with regard to the prevalence of coronary heart disease. Examples include a study from the Soviet Union[18] that found that 76 percent of men with coronary disease had high ratings on "strength of will, organizing abilities, ambition, and acceleration of rate of work" as opposed to 23 percent of controls. A Swedish paper found that women who had suffered myocardial infarctions "scored significantly higher than the healthy reference population on aggression, marginally higher on achievement, and significantly higher on a combined index called 'neurotic self-assertiveness' . . ."[19] A most inventive approach was taken by another researcher, who compared national mortality data from coronary disease in several countries with the rank ordering of the prominence of achievement themes in children's books from the same countries, and found a highly significant correlation.[20]

Several American studies over the years have established an association between the prevalence of coronary heart disease and of Type A behavior in a variety of populations, utilizing the Jenkins Activity Survey and the Structured Interview, as well as a number of lesser known tests for TABP[21-23] (for reviews see references 22, 24, and 25). Establishing mutual prevalence merely establishes the association between the two variables; it tells us nothing about how these variables interact or if any causality exists. Indeed, in looking at *prevalence* studies alone, one could surmise that coronary heart disease contributes to TABP instead of the intuitively more reasonable converse. Certainly it would be difficult to dispute such a hypothesis on the basis solely of prevalence data.

Incidence studies, which examine the incidence, or occurrence of a disease process over time, and hence are done prospectively, offer a more effective tool for examining dynamic interaction between variables. If we wish to establish that coronary heart disease develops more frequently in patients who display the TABP, we should first find a group of healthy individuals without clinical evidence of coronary heart disease whom we classify as Type A or B, and then follow them over time to ascertain who develops the illness. Note that no matter what the results of such studies are, we still cannot prove causality—but only infer it. We will, however, be much clearer about the evolution of coronary heart disease in Type A individuals, and thus have reason to intensify our search for the mechanism of the interaction so that we ultimately may better prevent and/or treat the disease.

Four major prospective studies deserve our attention in this context. The first, known as the Western Collaborative Group Study (WCGS), investigated 3154 initially well men aged 39–59. These men were examined for the presence of a number of risk factors, including TABP, and followed for eight and a half years. At the end of that time, 257 had developed coronary heart disease, and the men initially classified as Type A were seen to be 2.37 times more likely to be afflicted than those who were Type B. Type A as a completely independent risk factor produced a 1.97 times higher incidence. Therefore, other risk factors aside, the Type A individual had nearly twice the risk of developing coronary disease as did his Type B counterpart.[26]

The Framingham study, perhaps the most famous prospective cardiovascular investigation in history, was designed to study exhaustively the cardiovascular risks and subsequent development of disease among members of the community of Framingham, Mass. Its findings are far too lengthy to detail here, and have been the subject of numerous publications, but particularly relevant to our inquiry was the group of 1822 men and women administered a TABP questionnaire, which was similar to but far more comprehensive than the Jenkins Activity Survey. Some 148 of these individuals had clinical coronary heart disease at intake, and this correlated significantly with TABP prevalence. The remainder were followed for eight years, and as in the WCGS study, Type A men were found to be more than twice as likely to develop coronary heart disease as measured by the presence of angina or myocardial infarction than Type B men. The numbers for women were even more striking, with the incidence of infarction and angina 2.75 times more likely overall in Type A's.[27]

A subgroup of 269 couples from the Framingham population was administered an extensive questionnaire dealing with characteristics of their spouses, in addition to the other data gathered at intake. Ten years later their incidence of coronary heart disease was reviewed and correlated with psychosocial attributes of their marriages, as well as TABP, with the emergence of some rather interesting insights. Coronary risk was only significant in Type A men if their spouses (1) had more than 13 years of education (risk 2.5 times Type B) or (2) worked outside the home (3.5 times risk). The highest risks occurred in Type A men married to Type B women (25 percent coronary heart disease incidence) as compared with Type B/Type B couples (7.8 percent).[28] Other aspects of this subgroup are discussed in Chapter 5.

In another study 2437 Japanese males living in Hawaii were administered the Activity Survey and followed prospectively for coronary heart disease incidence. Men who both were Type A and had undergone some degree of cultural transformation by becoming more "westernized" were two to three times more likely to develop coronary heart disease than their peers.[29]

Finally, one major study that does not support the association of TABP and CHD was the study in which thousands of subscribers to the Kaiser-Permanente Health Plan in California completed a 155-item true–false questionnaire upon enrollment.[30] Items were selected from this questionnaire retrospectively as to whether they reflected Type A characteristics, and then compared with the incidence of coronary disease that subsequently had developed. None of these items were found to predict coronary heart disease. The weaknesses of the study include the unreliability of these items as predictors of TABP (they were not examined against a known instrument such as Activity Survey or the Structured Interview) and the wide range of ages studied (including patients over 70). Nonetheless, our "perfect" model has sprung a leak, albeit a small one.

It is important to note that Type B individuals are certainly not immune to coronary disease, in that other factors (e.g., smoking) are equal to or more powerful than behavior patterns in conferring risk, and that these risks operate independently.[27-31] We must also remind ourselves that Type A behavior is not an all-or-none phenomenon; it is possible that only certain components of TABP carry risk, and some of these components may be present in an otherwise Type B individual. We discuss this further shortly.

We have almost completed the first stage of our investigation into the association of TABP and coronary heart disease. What remains is to explore the relationship of the severity of coronary disease to the extent of TABP. In this context we will also be able to examine separate components of TABP and their relevance to coronary heart disease. This is most important, not only for our patients but because many health care providers are indeed Type A, in that is seems to be a frequent concomitant of success in Western society, and an apparent aid during the higher education process. It would be comforting to know, for those "A's" among us (which the writer would indeed classify himself), that not all components of the pattern confer risk.

In that the extent of coronary disease is best measured by coronary angiography, we are interested in research correlating angiographic findings with various measures of the TABP. Several studies deserve our attention. The first, done in 1976, compared results of the Activity Survey with catheterization data in 94 male patients.[32] It should be noted that this was not a random sample of the male population in that catheterization is associated with some risk and so undertaken only when clinical suspicion of disease is high. Thus it is likely that many of the men did have coronary heart disease. This suits our purposes, however, in that we are interested in the severity of the disease, not its presence or absence.

The study demonstrated that "the 55 men with 50 percent or

greater arterial obstruction in two or more vessels scored on the average statistically higher than the 36 with less disease on all four scales of the Jenkins Activity Survey." This study utilized a number of statistical techniques in an attempt to avoid confounding variables, and results remained significant when controlled for age, history of prior infarctions, or frequency of anginal episodes.

Two studies done in 1978[9,33] reported similar findings, with a few added twists. One, which used the Structured Interview to assess the TABP, looked at the other major risk factors simultaneously and found that the correlation of the TABP with severity of disease was of the same order of magnitude as other risk factors, with the exception of cholesterol, which was greater, and smoking and hypertension, which were less. It was found, moreover, that many of the Type B individuals catheterized had little if any disease, and that the findings held true for both sexes. The potency, then, of the TABP as a risk factor for coronary heart disease is as great or greater than some of the "classical" risks so universally accepted by medicine, at least according to this research. If such data are consistent, they should have at least some impact on our therapeutic endeavors.

The second study that year followed a similar protocol with quite definitive findings. These researchers were able to demonstrate the TABP among 44 percent of patients with mild disease, 69 percent with moderate occlusion, and 93 percent with severe coronary heart disease. This remained the case when other risk factors were controlled for. In addition, they found that individuals with elevated serum cholesterol were more likely to be Type A than those with normal values, a first link between two risk factors. Interestingly, this study utilized both the Activity Survey and the Structured Interview and only the latter measure of the TABP was found to be significant. The researchers attribute this discrepancy to the fact that their study population came from primarily rural environments and was of both sexes, whereas the Jenkins Activity Survey was originally standardized on an urban male population.

The finding in all of these studies that Type A behavior occurs at all levels of coronary disease, although it is statistically more prevalent with more severe occlusion, provides strong evidence against a hypothesis that we previously mentioned as being intuitively unlikely, namely, that the disease process of coronary heart disease produces the TABP, rather than the converse. In addition, as we discuss more extensively in the next chapter, Type A behavior is demonstrable in children and adolescents, who are almost certainly free of coronary heart disease.

Now, lest we be overwhelmed by the preponderance of evidence supporting the premise of Type A behavior as an independent risk factor for coronary disease, we must present some contrary data, which utilize the same "gold standard" of angiography. A study reported in 1983[34] failed to demonstrate any association between the severity of coronary heart disease and the presence of TABP using three different measures of the behavior, including the Structured Interview and two questionnaires somewhat similar to the Jenkins Activity Survey. Although the authors themselves seemed somewhat at a loss to explain their findings, their bias was evidenced in a rather interesting, though perhaps irrelevant, fashion. In support of their conclusions, they referred to three articles that described similar findings. Not only did one of these papers not support their findings, but it did not even address the issue; the other articles are discussed below. Another aspect of this research that is quite puzzling is the finding of a correlation between Type A behavior and *normal* exercise electrocardiograms. By contrast, Type B individuals were found to be more likely to display abnormal EKGs in response to treadmill testing, a finding totally unsupported in the medical literature. There is certainly no a priori reason why Type B patients should have a greater incidence of a finding generally indicative of coronary disease. The authors term this "uninterpretable."

The other two contradictory angiographic studies were performed by Dimsdale et al., using the Jenkins Activity Survey,[35] and the Structured Interview plus the Activity Survey[36] in separate populations of just over 100 patients each. In neither study was there seen a significant association between the Type A behavior pattern and coronary heart disease. The authors conclude:

> How can we explain the discrepancy between our findings and those of [similar studies]? The most likely explanation is that the samples studied in the three academic centers differ substantially on some relevant dimension. . . . Although we have no evidence about what this dimension may be, various psychosocial factors such as ethnicity, social class, stress and depression may well act to augment or dilute such a relationship.

Such work mandates that we not accept the premise of the

coronary heart disease/TABP interaction uncritically, but barring further research, I find the author's speculations concerning their contradictory work reasonable.

It is important to point out a potentially confounding factor in *all* of these studies: We do not know how the debilitating effects of symptomatic coronary heart disease influence the expression of the TABP. That is, does the presence of angina or a myocardial infarction modify a preexisting behavior pattern in some individuals, perhaps by inducing a blunting of joie de vivre, or a sense of hopelessness and resignation, the antithesis of Type A? Prevalence studies quoted earlier, which depended on symptomatic disease as a yardstick of coronary heart disease, and are overwhelming in their support of the hypothesis, would tend to contradict this idea, but cannot entirely invalidate it.

Perhaps some of the apparent contradictions result from a lack of sensitivity of the measuring tools for Type A traits in certain populations (see the discussion of correlation between Jenkins Activity Survey and Structured Interview) or the possibility that only certain Type A traits contribute to coronary risk.

Research already reviewed, and a few studies that we have not yet mentioned, have found certain components of the TABP to be more strongly associated with coronary heart disease than others. Some of the same studies that contradict the model found other behavioral characteristics that are significantly associated with coronary heart disease statistically independent of classic A/B typology, but that nonetheless seem related to the Type A trait.

One of the angiographic studies mentioned previously in support of the hypothesis found that the components of the TABP most significantly associated with coronary heart disease were aggressive content and an emphatic, rapid speech style. These were more significant than job commitment and time urgency, which when viewed in isolation were seen to be almost 50 percent less contributory to risk.[33]

The final trait receiving much current attention for its potential relationship to coronary heart disease is hostility. In 1980 a researcher, R. Williams, found a rather significant association between a measure of hostility called the Ho scale and the prevalence of coronary heart disease as diagnosed by angiography.[40] The difference in the severity of coronary disease between high- and low-scoring patients were marked, with 70 percent of those scoring above ten having greater than 75 percent narrowing of vessels, versus 48 percent of those with scores of less than ten. These findings were independent of TABP measurements, and in the minds of the researchers the trait represents an independent risk factor.

A second study[41] reported retrospectively an increased incidence of coronary heart disease based upon myocardial infarction or sudden (presumed cardiac) death in patients with high Ho scores measured 20 years previously. What is also interesting is that high hostility scores were associated with an overall 42 percent increased risk of death from *all* causes over the intervening 20 years. One other point of interest: The relationship of coronary heart disease to hostility was not linear; that is, though higher hostility scores are associated with an increased incidence of coronary heart disease, quantitatively more hostility after a certain point does not increase that risk.

A final study compared Ho scores obtained during routine psychological testing of a group of 255 medical students 25 years earlier with CHD and total mortality among the persons in that group as reported in 1983.[42] The same relationships were found to hold, again independently of other risk factors. Also, the overall increase in mortality in individuals with higher scores was again demonstrated.

Once again, the correlation between this candidate risk factor and components of the TABP is conceptually obvious (see Rosenman's definition of the TABP earlier in the chapter—the word hostility is not explicitly used, but synonyms abound). The Western Collaborative Group Study data were found to support the potential for hostility measured by the Structured Interview as related to CHD manifestations.[43] Here hostility was clearly considered part of the TABP. In another study both Structured Interview and Jenkins Activity Survey scores could be predicted by interviewer-judged hostility, among other traits.[44]

Table I, taken from Dembrowki et al.,[45] displays their correlations between components of the Type A pattern and overall Structured Interview interview typing in 50 male college students. Note particularly the high correlations between hostility and competitive behavior and the overall Type A score. (The closer the number is to 1.00, the higher is the correlation.)

Hence we who are Type A, or who work with Type A's, need

not assume that the trait in and of itself is the basis for the associated coronary disease risk; rather it may be a specific component or components of the pattern. Perhaps aggressiveness and hostility are the characteristics that put us at risk, a premise we consider later in the book.

If success in our society is desirable, then Type A behavior is clearly *not* all "bad," as demonstrated by the objective findings of greater achievement by Type A's. Type A social scientists were found to have a higher frequency of citations for meritorious scientific work than their Type B colleagues,[46] Jenkins Activity Survey scores correlated positively with course test scores in college students,[47] and Type A college students were found to be involved in more activities and to perform better scholastically than their Type B counterparts.[48]

Alas, the model is not perfect. The observed contradictions are perplexing, but, as we see throughout this book, are ubiquitous in all areas of clinical research. When a model makes intuitive sense, we become emotionally attached to it; we enjoy the conjunction of logic and sensibility; of rightness and reason. Therefore, we may feel distressed when confronted with contradiction, and hence develop biases that prevent objective interpretation. I certainly struggle with this. Nonetheless, the intuitive sensibility of this model, coupled with a preponderance of a variety of data supporting it, mandate in my mind a tentative acceptance of the concept coupled with a desire for more data, and a need to understand the contradictions.

Table 1. Intercorrelations Among Interview Stylistics and Content and Overall Interview Typing

	2	3	4	5	6	7	8
1. Loud and explosive	0.78	0.72	0.49	0.53	0.51	0.51	0.68
2. Rapid and accelerated		0.79	0.52	0.54	0.34	0.38	0.71
3. Response latency			0.57	:0.61	0.36	0.33	0.65
4. Hostility				0.76	0.40	0.50	0.68
5. Competition					0.34	0.40	0.73
6. Hard-driving content						0.57	0.46
7. Speed and impatience content							0.51
8. Overall interview typing							

Each reader must make this judgment independently. However, the model must advance an explanation for how the association of TABP and coronary heart disease might occur; we address this in the next chapter. There, also, we tie the knot between the stress response, TABP, and coronary heart disease. Let us close with the conclusions drawn by an illustrious panel of scientists & clinicians asked to review the data concerning the association of the Type A behavior pattern and coronary heart disease[31]:

> The review panel accepts the available body of evidence as demonstrating that Type A behavior—as defined by the Structured Interview, . . . the Jenkins Activity Survey, and the Framingham Type A behavior scale—is associated with an increased risk of clinically apparent CHD in employed, middle-aged U.S. citizens. This risk is greater than that imposed by age, elevated values of systolic blood pressure and serum cholesterol, and smoking, and appears to be of the same order of magnitude as the latter three factors.

REFERENCES

1. Van Dusch, T. *Lehrbuch der Herzkrankheiten.* Liepzig: Engelman, 1868.
2. Osler, W. The Lumleian lectures on angina pectoris. *Lancet,* 1:839–844, 1892.
3. Menninger, K. A., and Menninger, W. C. Psychoanalytic observations in cardiac disorders. *Am. Heart J,* 11:10–26, 1936.
4. Dunbar, H. F. *Psychosomatic Diagnosis.* New York: Hoeber, 1943.
5. Stewart, I. M. G. Coronary disease and modern stress. *Lancet,* 2:867–878, 1950.
6. Hancock, W. Coronary artery disease—Epidemiology and prevention. In E. Rubenstein, and D. Federman (eds.), *Scientific American Medicine.* New York: Scientific American, 1982.
7. Rosenman, R., and Chesney, M. A., Stress, Type A behavior, and coronary disease. In L. Goldberger and S. Breznitz (eds.), *Handbook of Stress: Theoretical and Clinical Aspects.* New York: Macmillan, 1982.
8. Rosenman, R. The interview method of asessment of the coronary-prone behavior pattern. In Dembrowski et al. (eds.), *Coronary-Prone Behavior.* New York: Springer-Verlag, 1978.
9. Blumenthal, J. A., Wiliams, R., Kong, Y., et al, Type A behavior pattern and coronary atherosclerosis. *Circulation,* 58:634–639, 1978.
10. Jenkins, C. D., Rosenman, R., and Friedman, M. Development of an objective psychological test for the determination of the coronary-prone behavior pattern in employed men. *J Chron Dis,* 20:371–379, 1967.
11. Brunson, B., and Matthews, K. The Type A coronary-prone behavior pattern and reactions to uncontrollable stress: An analysis of performance strategies, affect, and attributions during failure. *J Per Soc Psychol,* 40:906–918, 1981.
12. Pittner, M. S., and Houston, K. Response to stress, cognitive coping strategies, and the Type A behavior pattern. *J Pers Soc Psychol,* 39:147–157, 1980.

13. Blumenthal, J. A., et al. Effect of task incentive on cardiovascular response in type A and Type B individuals. *Psychophysiology*, 20:63–69, 1938.
14. Dembrowski, T. M., Macdougall, J., et al. Effect of level of challenge on pressor and heart rate responses in Type A and B subjects. *J Appl Soc Psychol*, 9:209–228, 1979.
15. Brand, R. J., Rosenman, R. H., Jenkins, C. D., et al. Comparison of coronary heart disease prediction in the Western Collaborative Group Study using the Structured Interview and the Jenkins Activity Survey assessments of the coronary-prone type A behavior pattern. Unpublished manuscript, University of California, Berkeley, 1978.
16. Zyzanski, S. J., Wrzesniewski, K., and Jenkins, C. D. Cross cultural validation of the coronary-prone behavior pattern. *Soc Sci Med*, 13A:405–412, 1979.
17. Kittel, F., Kornitzer, M., Zyzanski, S. J., et al. Two methods of assessing the coronary-prone behavior pattern in Belgium. *J Chron Dis*, 31:147–155, 1978.
18. Ganelina, I. E., and Kraevsky, Y. M. Premorbid personality peculiarities in patients with cardiac ischemia. *Kardiologiia*, 11:40–55, 1971. As reviewed in Jenkins, C. D. Recent evidence supporting psychologic and social risk factors for coronary disease, part 2. *N Engl J Med*, 294:1033–1038, 1976.
19. Bengtsson, C., Hallstrom, T., and Tibbin, G. Social factors, stress experience, and personality traits in women with ischaemic heart disease, compared to a population sample of women. *Acta Med Scand* [Suppl]549:82–92, 1973. Reviewed in Jenkins, C.D., *Ibid*.
20. Appels, A. Het hartinfarct een cultuurziekte. *Tijdschr Soc Geneek* 50:446–448, 1972. Reviewed in Jenkins, C. D., *Ibid*.
21. Jenkins, C. D., Zyzanski, S. J., Rosenman, R. H., et al. Association of coronary-prone behavior scores with recurrence of coronary heart disease. *J Chron Dis*, 24:601–611, 1971.
22. Rosenman, R. H., and Chesney, M. A. The relationship of Type A behavior pattern to coronary heart disease. *Act Nerv Sup*, 22:1–45, 1980.
23. Friedman, M., and Rosenman, R. H. Association of specific, overt behavior pattern with blood and cardiovascular findings. *JAMA*, 169:1286–1296, 1959.
24. Feinlieb, M., Brand, R. J., Remington, R., and Zyzanski, S. J. Association of the coronary-prone behavior pattern and coronary heart disease. In S. M. Dembrowski, et al. (eds.), *Coronary-Prone Behavior* New York: Springer, 1978.
25. Jenkins, C. D. Recent evidence supporting psychologic and social risk factors for coronary disease. *N Engl J Med*, 294:1033–1038, 1976.
26. Rosenman, R. H., Brand, R. J., et al. Multivariate prediction of coronary heart disease in the Western Collaborative Group Study: Final followup of 8 1/2 years. *JAMA*, 37:903–910, 1975.
27. Haynes, S. G., Feinlieb, M., and Kannel, W. B. The relationship of psychosocial factors to coronary disease in the Framingham Study. Part III: Eight year incidence of CHD. *Am J Epidemiol*, 3:37–58, 1980.
28. Eaker, E. D., Haynes, S. G., and Feinlieb, M. Spouse behavior and coronary heart disease in men: Prospective results from the Framingham Heart Study. II. Modification of risk in Type A husbands according to the social and psychological status of their wives. *Am J Epidemiol*, 118:23–41, 1983.
29. Cohen, J. B., Syme, S. L., Jenkins, C. D., et al. The cultural context of Type A behavior and the risk of CHD. *Am J Epidemiol*, 102:434, 1975.

30. Friedman, G. D., Ury, H. K., Klatsky, A. L., et al. A psychological questionnaire predictive of myocardial infarction: Results from the Kaiser-Permanente Epidemiologic Study of Myocardial Infarction. *Psychosom Med,* 36:327–343, 1974.
31. The Review Panel on Coronary-Prone Behavior and Coronary Heart Disease. Coronary-prone behavior and coronary heart disease: A critical review. *Circulation,* 63:1199–1215, 1981.
32. Zyzanski, S., Jenkins, C. D., Ryan, T. J., et al. Psychological correlates of coronary angiographic findings. *Arch Intern Med,* 136:1234–1237, 1976.
33. Frank, K., Heller, S., Kornfeld, D., et al. Type A behavior pattern and coronary angiographic findings. *JAMA,* 240:761–763, 1978.
34. Scherwitz, L., McKelvain, R., and Laman, C. Type A behavior, self-involvement, and coronary atherosclerosis. *Psychosom Med* 45:47–57, 1983.
35. Dimsdale, J. E., Hackett, T., and Hutter, A. M. Type A personality and extent of coronary atherosclerosis. *Am J Cardiol,* 42:583–586, 1978.
36. Dimsdale, J., Hutter, A. M., Block, P. et al. Type A behavior and angiographic findings. *J Psychosom Res,* 23:273–276, 1979.
37. Scheier, M., and Carver, C. Focused self attention and the experience of emotion: attraction, repulsion, elation, and depression. *J Pers Soc Psychol,* 35:625–636, 1977. As referenced in 34.
38. Carver, C. Facilitation of aggression through objective self-awareness. *Exp Soc Psychol,* 10:365–370, 1974. As referenced in 34.
39. Weintraub, W. *Verbal Behavior: Adaptation and Psychopathology.* New York: Springer, 1981. As referenced in 34.
40. Williams, R., Haney T., Lee, K., et al. Type A behavior, hostility, and coronary heart disease. *Psychosom Med,* 42: 539–549, 1980.
41. Shekelle, R. B., Gale, M., Ostfeld, A., and Oglesby, P. Hostility, risk of coronary heart disease, and mortality. *Psychosom Med,* 45:109–114, 1983.
42. Barefoot, J. C., Dahlstrom, W. G., and Williams, R. B. Hostility, CHD incidence, and total mortality: A 25-year follow-up study of 255 physicians. *Psychosom Med,* 45:59–63, 1983.
43. Matthews, K., Glass, D., Rosenman, R., et al. Competitive drive, pattern A and coronary heart disease: A further analysis of some data from the Western Collaborative Group Study. *J Chron Dis,* 30:489–498, 1977.
44. Matthews, K. A., Krantz, D. S., Dembrowski, T. M., and MacDougall, J. M. Unique and common variance in structured interview and Jenkins Activity Survey measurements of the Type A behavior pattern. *J Pers Soc Psychol,* 42:303–313, 1982.
45. Dembrowski, T. M., MacDougall, J. M., et al. Components of the Type A coronaryprone behavior pattern and cardiovascular responses to psychomotor performance challenge. *J Behav Med* 1:159–176, 1978.
46. Matthews, K. A., Heimreich, R. L., Beane, W. E., et al. Pattern A, achievement striving, and scientific merit: Does pattern A help or hinder? *J Pers Soc Psychol,* 39:962–967, 1980.
47. Becker, M. A., and Suls, J. Test performance as a function of the hard-driving and speed components of the Type A coronary-prone behavior pattern. *J Psychosom Res,* 26:435–440, 1982.
48. Ovcharchyn, C. A., Johnson, H. H., and Petzel, T. P. Type A behavior, academic aspirations, and academic success. *J Pers,* 49:248–256, 1981.

4

GETTING AHEAD: HURRYING, HOSTILITY, AND HYPERREACTIVITY

*T*he association between the Type A behavior pattern (TABP) and coronary heart disease was a landmark finding in medicine, despite the reticence of some to accept its validity. The finding is unique in that it was the first of its kind to demonstrate a link between a specific psychogenic process and an organic disease. As such, I find it fascinating that most contemporary medical textbooks either ignore the subject, or treat it in a terse sentence or so. This is particularly disturbing in light of the fact that the risk for developing coronary disease if one possesses the Type A pattern is at least of the same order of magnitude as the other "classical" risk factors.

Medical training is often relatively bereft of considerations of the psyche, and consequently most clinicians are generally uncomfortable with, unlearned about, and unskilled in the diagnosis and therapy of such disorders. They find it much easier to tell a patient to stop smoking, to prescribe therapy for hypertension, or to suggest a diet for hyperlipidemia than to diagnose and treat a disorder whose roots are muddy, whose interventions are poorly defined, and whose characteristics they frequently share. The time alone involved in these approaches is prohibitive for most doctors today, unless they are psychiatrists.

Consequently, the assessment and therapy for this element of coronary risk fall to so-called "ancillary medical personnel," perhaps such as you, the reader. One should not expect much support from physicians in the way of suggestions regarding this dimension of health, but a sound knowledge of the literature and the mechanisms involved will go a long way toward establishing the validity of the psychosomatic premise, and convincing clinicians of the importance of the TABP.

Nonetheless, an epidemiologic reality has been defined, and will not disappear by being ignored. In the next several chapters, we investigate the physiology of the TABP—we look to its roots, development, environmental triggers, and pathologic impact on the heart and vasculature. We demonstrate its often dramatic effect on patients with estasblished coronary disease, what risks these patients face, and what can be done to intervene. We explore the "symptoms" of unfavorable impact on the organism, whether self-recognition of the TABP is reliable, and what modalities of therapy hold a promise of efficacy in reducing risk. We then propose some concrete programs in this regard. It is my hope that clinicians as well might find herein a mandate for further research and self-education,

A model that appears promising for understanding the CHD-TABP interaction, and one upon which large parts of this book are based, is the stressor–stress response concept.

We postulated, in Chapters 1 and 2, a model of stress-induced disease—a pathologic effect of a sustained or repetitive stress response. It is relatively easy to induce illness in experimental animals by overcrowding them, introducing abnormal or unusual social situations, isolating them, or repeatedly applying noxious stimuli.

Diseases in experimental animals, however, have little ecological reality; they are artifacts of laboratory manipulation, and probably do not occur to any significant degree in free-living animal populations. But the problem of coronary heart disease *is* an ecological one: The disease certainly does occur in free-living human populations. What are the interactions between humans and their environment that create this disease? As with any ecological problem, the answer is multifactorial. We established in the last chapter that one of these factors, operating independently, is a behavioral characteristic—a way of coping with environmental stressors. Let us postulate that the TABP is the behavioral analog of one of our familiar stress responses: sympathomedullary arousal, or "fight or flight." Further, let us hypothesize that the impact of the TABP on heart disease is via this stress response.

In this chapter we investigate this hypothesis and its implications.

Our investigation again proceeds by stages. We first address the question of whether the TABP might actually represent a true stress response. In the past we have discussed stress responses as organic processes involving hormones and nerves. It is indeed possible (and likely) that such responses are accompanied by affective or behavioral phenomena (such as fighting or fleeing), and perhaps the TABP is one such external manifestation. We will therefore investigate physiologic reactions accompanying TABP. We have already indicated that the TABP is evoked: We will inquire as to which environmental elements are most potent in eliciting this behavior, and whether such elements are capable of acting as true stressors.

We next look at various populations of Type A individuals, including children, and investigate the nature and intensity of their stress responses. We also inquire as to whether such responses are solely the province of Type A individuals, and whether they are present in patients with established coronary disease. All of this will be interwoven into a model of TABP, stress, and coronary disease.

We earlier described a stress response characterized by the outpouring of adrenaline (epinephrine) and activation of the sympathetic nervous system in response to perceived challenge or threat (see Chapter 2). The function of this fight-or-flight response is to create a state of physiologic arousal that "enables" the organism—that is, prepares it—to deal with physical threat. This state of sympathomedullary arousal consists of increases in heart rate and the force of cardiac contraction; redistribution of blood away from the skin and gastrointestinal tract and to skeletal muscle, heart, and lungs; dilation of the airways and pupils; and high levels of sensory awareness. The utility of many of these changes in a physical threat situation is obvious. It is not clear, however, that a response of this nature to contemporary challenges in a civilized environment is adaptive, and could be deleterious. Indeed, it has been postulated that such a stress response, triggered inappropriately in the face of nonphysical threat, could lead to damage to the target organs of "sympathomedullary arousal," namely, the heart and vasculature. We examine this premise in detail shortly.

It is appropriate to inquire first whether such a stress response is a feature of human reactions to psychogenic stimuli, who displays such reactivity, and under what circumstances. A logical starting place is the Type A individual, whom we have already defined as responding to environmental stimuli in a rather aroused mode behaviorally. Let us seek physiologic analogs.

Quite early in the exploration of the Type A phenomenon, it was suggested that physiologic hyperresponsiveness might accompany the behavior pattern. A paper was published in 1960 that measured urine concentrations of the hormones epinephrine and norepinephrine in Type A and Type B men both during working hours and at night[1] The finding that Type A men secreted "far more norepinephrine" during working hours than their Type B counterparts whereas nighttime secretions did not differ was not surprising to the researchers; they were already aware that TABP is an evoked phenomenon, and accompanying metabolic changes should, they reasoned, follow suit.

Though previous research had demonstrated increased catecholamine (the generic term for epinephrine and norepinephrine) secretion in emotionally stressful situations,[2,3] this was the first attempt to elucidate a physiologic concomitant to the TABP. As demonstrated in Chapter 2, the catecholamines are the prime mediators of the fight-or-flight stress response.

An eloquent model begins to evolve. TABP is the external manifestation of catecholamine storm induced by environmental stressors, and with its hostility, time urgency, and competitive components, it is behaviorally suited to optimize the organism's response to external threat. Coronary disease occurs because contemporary stressors are psychological, no longer requiring physical responsiveness, and the catecholamines arouse a sedentary heart and vasculature, which are not called upon to pump blood to flailing arms or running legs. The storm is bottled up and vents its fury on the bottle.

An interesting, eminently sensible hypothesis that has received much support over the ensuing years, the "cardiovascular hyperreactivity" theory, may indicate the mechanism for the CHD-TABP interaction. Let us take a closer look.

Studies have approached the issue from one or both of two basic perspectives: biochemical, involving measurement of blood or urine catecholamines; and physiologic, or measuring catecholamine effects on the body as an index of their presence. The latter includes measurements of blood pressure, heart rate, electrocardiographic changes, forearm blood flow, and finger pulse amplitude, and similar, generally noninvasive measures designed to assess catecholamine effects on the body. These measurements are all reflections, of greater or lesser accuracy, of the impact of catecholamines on their target organs.

Regardless of the measurements taken, the basic design of most of these studies involves applying a laboratory stressor (a contrived, controlled situation) to Type A and B individuals, and measuring sympathomedullary arousal by one or more of these methods.

The information obtained is not limited to the differences in arousal between Type A's and B's, but also helps to elucidate the nature of the stressors capable of such arousal and their relative potency in doing so. By examining such work carefully, we may learn much about the pathogenesis of the catecholamine stress response and how it interacts with the TABP.

A key question about differential reactivity between A's and B's is whether such differences, if they exist, are caused by exposure to different conditions in their respective environments, thus requiring different responses, or by different responses to identical stimuli. An attempt to answer this question in a more rigorous fashion than the 1960 study was undertaken by the same group 15 years later, by "standardizing" the environment.[4] They subjected 15 clinically well Type A males and the same number of Type B's to a challenging puzzle whose solution was "of little intrinsic importance." A reward of excellent French wine was offered to the winner, but the puzzle was unsolvable. "Irritating" rock-and-roll music was played on two different stations simultaneously to enhance the stress of the situation. Blood was drawn repeatedly for catecholamine determinations during the study.

Behaviorly, the differences between the groups were obvious at the outset, during pretest instructions, with the Type A individuals "tense, hyperalert, and impatient," and the B's "relaxed and even amused." Furthermore, during the challenge itself:

> The majority of [the Type A] subjects competitively attempted solution of the puzzle almost as if their lives depended on the outcome. Even after the contest was declared over, the augmented intensity and pitch of their voices and the abrupt and hyperkinetic style of their various motor activities made

it obvious that the Type A individuals had overreacted to the stimulus presented to them, as compared with the reactions of Type B subjects.

This is not surprising, nor is the fact that the Type A individuals had significantly higher pretest norepinephrine values than the Type B subjects, and increased these values significantly in response to the challenge. What lends further weight to the hypothesis is that the Type B values did not change in response to challenge, nor was *any* difference between baseline A and B values shown in a non-challenge situation presented at another time!

Notice that this study was clearly designed to elicit Type A behavior by presenting a challenging problem and stimulating competition. Both groups were exposed to the same stimulus, yet the Type A's were more profoundly aroused, both behaviorally and biochemically.

A number of other studies, seeking to explore nuances of these findings, have investigated the responses of Type A's to an array of laboratory stressors, in an attempt to sort out those components of stress most potent in eliciting hyperreactivity. Most of these studies have looked at physiologic, as opposed to biochemical, parameters on the assumptions that (1) increased levels of circulating catecholamines affect target organs (heart, blood vessels) in a predictable, measurable fashion, and (2) any pathologic consequences of the stress response are likely to result from effects on these organs. Hence the studies we are about to discuss have used variations on a theme of "electrophysiologic monitoring," ranging from dynamic measurements of heart rate, blood pressure, and blood flow to fingertips and forearms to observations of electrocardiographic changes and pulse transit times (the faster the pulse of blood is propagated through the body, the greater the catecholamine stimulation of the heart is felt to be). None of these techniques is universally accepted as an accurate reflection of circulating catecholamines; however, each has a theoretical basis for validity, is generally reproducible, and is noninvasive (i.e., does not require needle puncture), and when they are correlated with each other, probably are reasonable yardsticks of cardiovascular arousal. (For a detailed discussion of electrophysiologic methodology, see reference 5.) Where relevant in subsequent discussions, we address weak points in methodologies or assumptions made by researchers in this regard.

A study that measured blood pressure and heart rate changes as indices of cardiovascular arousal in response to a difficult cognitive task demonstrated a clear difference between Type A and B males, with the A's responding to the challenge with greater blood pressure increases[6]. The test was administered under time-constraint conditions with small monetary rewards for correct performance. An important finding (the implications of which we discuss later) was a lack of such differences between Type A and B females. Once again the experimental conditions were designed specifically to elicit Type A behavior. Similar findings were obtained in two other studies measuring the same physiologic parameters in response to challenges to performance at "TV handball"[7] and problem-solving skills.[8]

Although the methodologies differ, the above studies have in common the finding that under TABP-provoking circumstances, a clear difference exists between the cardiovascular reactivity of male Type A and B subjects. Next we might inquire as to what *types* of stress are necessary to elicit the observed differences (i.e., performance challenge, physical versus psychological stressors, threats to self-esteem versus physical pain) and which are the most potent in eliciting hyperreactivity.

Research has indeed been performed comparing reactivity with physical and cognitive challenge in A's versus B's.[9,10,36]

Though the data are not overwhelming, these papers agree that Type A males appear somewhat more reactive than Type B's to challenging laboratory stressors, particularly when imposed challenges are relevant to the TABP. The most reactive individuals were A's in a high-challenge situation. However, the challenge component was not a prerequisite for A's to react; rather the task itself was all that was necessary. There is evidence that Type A's may be more reactive to physical stressors as well.[36] The trend for Type A's to be the most reactive under high challenge conditions is reasonably consistent across both psychologic and physical stressors, but clearly A's respond to the task itself without requiring explicit prodding. It would seem that challenge may have been implicit in the above studies, at least to A's, whether or not it was explicitly stated.

A variation on the theme is suggested: If there truly *is* no challenge to the task, is the *belief* in challenge adequate to stimulate arousal?

This was studied in 1981 by Gastorf,[13] who set up an experimental situation involving tasks that were easy or hard, presented with instructions that implied the tasks were easy or hard. Hence some subjects took easy tests they expected to be difficult, some took difficult tests they expected to be easy, and others took tests whose instructions correctly matched their difficulty.

Type A's demonstrated greater arousal than B's with regard to both the hard task they expected to be hard and the hard task they expected to be easy. Type B's did become aroused (although not to the same level as A's) to a hard task they expected to be hard. Type A's were also more significantly aroused than B's when confronted with an easy test they expected to be hard. Interesting and enlightening was the lack of arousal demonstrated by both A's and B's to an easy task expected to be easy.

It would seem from this work that subjective and objective challenges are equipotent at eliciting arousal in Type A individuals, but truly low-challenge conditions presented without explicit challenge instructions do not provoke reactivity. Hence not all circumstances are accompanied by hyperresponsiveness, and both expectation and reality of challenge play a role in defining the Type A's physiology.

Other stressors in addition to performance challenge probably are capable of eliciting physiologic arousal. Certainly, in an evolutionary sense, threatening circumstances would be expected to do so, yet only one study specifically compares A's and B's in reponse to a threat.[14]

Two distinct types were studied: threat to self-esteem and threat of electric shock. Challenges to self-esteem were far more physiologically arousing than physical threat, at least in the group of college students tested. There were significant interpretive flaws in this work, however, that cloud my view of the results.

A final component of the stressor potency issue is the effect of task incentive on cardiovascular reactivity. The dimension of incentive is a motivational one as opposed to challenging or threatening circumstances that are not associated with significant positive rewards for success. One might hypothesize that the Type A's would be more hyperreactive than B's in an incentive condition, because of a relationship to the TABP construct. However, this is not the case. In A's reactivity was present to the challenges presented in two studies[15,16] regardless of incentive.

Many studies of this nature are tedious to review and difficult to interpret, with conclusions sometimes drawn on marginal data. Frequently the physiologic variables studied do not agree, and the meaning and significance of these variables are endlessly debated.[17,18] Nonetheless we may present some general conclusions that can be drawn with, I believe, some validity at this stage in our investigation.

1. There appear to be no differences in physiologic states as they relate to sympathomedullary arousal between Type A and B males and females at rest (a virtually universal finding in all of the reviewed research).
2. Type A males are generally more cardiovascularly responsive than Type Bs to laboratory challenges or stressors, particularly when they are relevant to the TABP construct, involving challenge, time urgency, or threat to self-esteem.
3. Type A males are variably more hyperreactive to physical stressors than Type B's, particularly when an element of challenge is involved.
4. Challenge need not be real, but only perceptual, to evoke reactivity in A's.
5. Physical threat is not as potent as psychological threat in eliciting hyperreactivity.
6. Task incentive is not a potent force in eliciting sympathomedullary arousal in A's, though it may be in B's.

Before moving on to the link between TABP, cardiovascular hyperreactivity, and coronary disease, we need to address our two other questions: (1) Are specific components of the Type A pattern more prone to cardiovascular arousal than others? (2) Are there significant sex differences? We also briefly explore the TABP and arousal in children, and then turn our attention to coronary heart disease.

Recall from the last chapter the greater reliability of hostility and competitiveness components of the TABP in predicting coronary heart disease than the behavior pattern as a whole. One would, therefore, expect that if cardiovascular arousal is an important mechanism in the pathogenesis of coronary heart disease, these components ought to be associated with greater reactivity. This issue was specifically addressed in the study by Theodore Dembrowki.[7] The data demonstrated that hostility as measured by Structured Interview stylistics was the most strongly predictive of physiologic arousal, followed by "rapid accelerated speech and verbal competitiveness." Other components, including impatience, speed, and hard-driving behaviors, were less clear-cut, and varied in their correlations, depending on whether Structured Interview or Jenkins Activity Survey criteria were used.

Earlier we discussed another study by Dembrowski[9], in which he attempted to determine whether a challenge variable was relevant to Type A hyperreactivity. Recall that was so, but the data were not overwhelming, and A's reacted to an experimental situation whether or not they were challenged. However, an additional finding of that study was that Type A-highly hostile individuals were hyperreactive across both challenge conditions, for both physical and psychological stressors, whereas the Type A less hostile individuals were hyperreactive only in the high-challenge state. In fact, the latter individuals more closely resembled Type B's in their responsiveness. This global hyperreactivity in hostile Type A's may explain the lack of effect of the challenge variable noted when all A's are lumped together. The implications of global reactivity in coronary heart disease pathogenesis may be profound, as we shall discuss. Hostility, that least desirable of the Type A traits, again demonstrates its detrimental effects on human physiology.

Most of the studies cited thus far have involved male subjects. Coronary disease is certainly not an exclusively male affliction, however, it is well known that women are relatively immune to the disease until after menopause. The reasons for this are unclear, but generally felt to be hormonally related. It *is* clear that following menopause women catch up rapidly, and the same risk factors appear to be operative. We also know from the last chapter that Type A behavior in women is associated with an increased incidence of coronary disease. Hence one might expect that studies in women would parallel findings in men. Alas, the situation is muddier than that.

Manuck et al.,[6] Lane et al.,[19] and MacDougall et al.[20] failed to demonstrate differences in physiologic arousal in A and B females to challenges similar in design to work on males, including cold pressor and reaction-time tests, as well as forced mental arithmetic. Just as the puzzle begins to assemble itself coherently, the pieces are swept off the table. Need we be so dramatic? Well it does seems that if cardiovascular hyperreactivity is to attain candidacy as a mechanism linking the TABP and Coronary Heart Disease, a major inconsistency such as this could be fatal.

Fortunately there are some feasible explanations for these findings. All of the foregoing studies utilized female undergraduate students between the ages of 18 and 22. Perhaps young women have not yet developed the capacity for cardiovascular hyperreactivity to laboratory stressors, a capability which manifests itself more fully in later years. We have some support from the literature for this contention. A study of differential catecholamine release in response to a color conflict test that compared "young" (22–34-year-old) females and males with "older" (ages 50–67) individuals found: "Adrenaline secretion increased markedly in all but the young female group as an effect of the color conflict test."[21]

Young females did, however, show increases in heart rate and skin conductance levels in response to the stressors, which is somewhat hard to reconcile with the biochemical findings.

An alternative, and not mutually exclusive, explanation for the foregoing is that young women possess fewer Type A traits, but these increase with age. An interesting study by Waldron et al.[24] seems to support this, in that in an 18–25-year-old group, male Jenkins Activity Study scores were significantly higher than those for females, whereas in the 26–44-year-old population, they were virtually identical. In the following year, Waldron[25] went on to show that working women with some college education in the 40–59-year-old age group were significantly more Type A than their nonworking or working non-college-educated contemporaries. So it seems that age, education, and employment status may play significant roles in defining the Type A female. We return to this concept at the end of the chapter. To bolster our contention that the Type A behavior/CHD interaction in women is mediated by cardiovascular hyperreactivity, it would be useful to demonstraste this reactivity in older Type A females.

Data unfortunately are scanty, but one recent study specifically addresses this point[26]. Lawler et al. tested a mixed group of 41 women aged 25–55 for physiologic responsiveness at rest and in response to mathematics and visual problem solving. Half the group were housewives; the others were professionals or executives. All were administered the Jenkins Activity Survey. Several observations and revelations emerged: (1) Ninety percent of employed females were strong Type A's. (2) Most unemployed Type A's indicated a strong desire for employment. (3) Type A women were significantly more reactive than B's. (4) Even among unemployed women, the Type A's were significantly more responsive physiologically than B's. So it seems, at least preliminarily, that Type A women over the age of 25 are cardiovascular hyperreactors to laboratory stressors, and this may well be a function of age.

Of course, the next questions that suggest themselves are: Can children be classified as A or B? Are the A's hyperreactive? Are there sex differences? The answers: yes, perhaps, and unclear. A good deal has been written about the TABP in children, and several measures of such behavior have been developed and tested. It seems that certain children do display the A characteristics of impatience, time urgency, competitiveness, anger, and hostility. The instruments by which such traits are measured are quite varied[27] and their validity debated, however, one study that utilized a modified Structured Interview[28] commented on the fact that the behavior seemed far more situation dependent than in adults. Perhaps this speaks to a situation-specific behavior in children that evolves into a relatively nonspecific response in adults, an issue to which we also return.

With regard to the issues of hyperreactivity and sex differences in children, the few studies available are contradictory and use different measures of the TABP. One study demonstrates greater reactivity in Type A boys aged three to six than in their B counterparts in response to physical challenge.[29] Another demonstrated this finding for 11–12-year-old girls, but not boys, for one measurement of the TABP, and for both sexes using a different assessment of the behavior.[30] This latter study acknowledged its limitations in the author's conclusions:

> The MYTH [a tool used in this work to measure the TABP in children] is not sufficiently precise to select Type A behavior in children.
> Our sample size was too small given instrument precision. Our tasks were inappropriate to elicit differences in the physiological responses of Type A and Type B individuals.

Such admissions of limitation are often helpful in placing results of scientific research in perspective, but are found all too rarely. All studies must be examined in terms of the restricted applicability of the results. Broad generalizations based on small sample sizes and selected populations are misleading and can be dangerous. It seems evident that there are insufficient data and too much variability in technique and methodology to make meaningful statements about the TABP and cardiovascular reactivity in children.

In summary, then, we might say that the Type A behavior pattern appears to be associated with a phenomenon of cardiovascular reactivity to environmental challenges, primarily those relevant to the behavior pattern. The phenomenon appears to be mediated via sympathetic nervous stimulation and the release of adrenaline from the adrenal medulla, and as such might be termed a physiologic stress response. Harkening back to our Chapter 1 definitions, we might, with reasonable validity, term the environmental challenges chronic intermittent stressors and sympathomedullary arousal the stress response. This stressor–stress response interaction would seem to be a likely candidate as the primary mediator between the TABP and CHD.

It would be useful to know whether cardiovascular hyperreactivity is a characteristic shared by patients with Coronary Heart Disease. Certainly we would expect to find that among patients with Coronary Heart Disease, Type A individuals are more hyperresponsive than B's (unless the disease process itself attenuates the phenomenon) and such a finding would lend weight to the contention that the pathogenic feature of the Type A pattern that renders it a Coronary Heart Disease risk *is* hyperreactivity.

Some very compelling evidence for cardiovascular hyperreactivity in Type A patients with coronary disease was presented in two different studies, both of which evaluated responsiveness of Coronary Heart Disease patients under stressful circumstances. What is so unique and startling about both of these papers was not the finding of hyperreactivity in Type A as opposed to B patients, but that this finding occurred during surgery under general anesthesia! Both research teams[31,32] studied groups of patients undergoing coronary bypass surgery, the process of grafting a vein to a clogged artery to bypass the blockage. Both groups, operating independently, found significant correlations between Type A ratings and extent of blood pressure rise during surgery. In addition, the more recent of the two[32] demonstrated that certain complications of surgery, felt generally to be a function of overactivity of the sympathetic nervous system, occurred only in Type A patients. We shall have much more to say about this point in the next chapter, when we deal with the pathologic effects of sympathomedullary arousal and the link to coronary disease.

What these papers demonstrate quite convincingly is the fact that Type A patients with Coronary Heart Disease (note this qualifier) need not be conscious to be physiologically aroused to a greater extent than their Type B counterparts when experiencing the same stressor. We saw a suggestion that this might be true in previously quoted work that demonstrated A's hyperresponsiveness to a physical stressor, but the bulk of evidence had it that conscious mediation and perception of stressors played an important role in eliciting arousal. The authors speculate: "Among these middle-aged patients there is an underlying biological or psychobiological factor (e.g., early conditioning of sympathoadrenomedullary responses) which mediates both the expression of Type A behavior and the link between Type A and coronary disease."[32]

What the authors seem to be suggesting is that Type A behavior is a concomitant of sympathetic nervous and adrenal activity, and hence it is itself a marker of arousal, an outward manifestation of innate processes requiring no conscious mediation, rather than their cause.[21]

There are few additional studies on physiologic arousal to stress in patients with Coronary Heart Disease. One, by Dembrowsi's group,[8] compared reactivity among and between four groups: Type A/Coronary Heart Disease, Type B/Coronary Heart Disease, Type A/no Coronary Heart Disease, and Type B/no Coronary Heart Disease. Sixty-four subjects were studied; all were middle-aged males. Again as expected, the Type A Coronary Heart Disease and no Coronary Heart Disease individuals were globally more reactive than their B counterparts. A fascinating and unexpected finding was that B/Coronary Heart Disease patients were equally as hyperreactive to an American history quiz as the A's, and this differed significantly from B/no Coronary Heart Disease. One might be led to speculate that Coronary Heart Disease itself may be associated with hyperreactivity—a finding of great potential significance, as we will see.

A further finding that should not be too surprising was that within the Type A sample, both hostility and competitive drive were significantly related to blood pressure increases.

Let me point out again that failure of an investigator properly to peruse the literature of a subject renders the findings somewhat suspect with regard to their validity. In this case, despite the intriguing findings, I view the study somewhat skeptically because of a misinterpretation of a previous paper we have already discussed[2] that the authors used to bolster the validity of their findings. The authors specifically state:

> The results are also consistent with the finding[2] that both coronary symptom-free Type A subjects and coronary patients showed significant elevations in norepinephrine during a competitive contest, while Type B subjects engaged in the same contest displayed no such changes in catecholamine levels.

This is exciting, if true. We have mentioned that there is a paucity of information on the subject. Unfortunately the authors of the referenced article specifically state: "All Type A and B subjects were normotensive and appeared free of coronary disease as judged by the absence of all cardiovascular symptoms, and the exhibition of normal electrocardiograms." The paper was explicitly designed to study "clinically normal" subjects; no patients with Coronary Heart Disease were included.

Perhaps this is nit-picking. Nonetheless, when important conclusions must be tentatively based on only a few studies, the accuracy of the research is critical, and I initially regarded this study with some reservation.

Fortunately for the authors, two subsequent studies supported their findings, namely, that as a group, CHD patients are more reactive than non-coronary disease individuals, and in some instances, virtually independent of A/B typology.[33,34]

What do we do with a finding that coronary heart disease patients may be hyperreactors independent of A/B typology? This could suggest that Type A behavior is not the only marker for sympathomedullary arousal, and that the entire coronary heart disease/Type A interaction only hints at a far broader interaction between psyche and soma.

Let me elaborate. If patients with coronary heart disease who are also Type B are hyperreactors, then one might hypothesize that the final common denominator between coronary heart disease and psychosocial stress is sympathomedullary arousal irrespective of A/B typology. The TABP becomes an external marker of reactivity only in certain individuals who in essence demonstrate a behavioral correlate of reactivity. Above and beyond those individuals might be a population of non-A's who, despite an absence of behavioral manifestations, react physiologically to environmental stressors—individuals we might term "silent reactors." If this were the case, we would find it necessary to develop new methods of identifying individuals at risk, and not feel very protected by being classified as Type B behaviorally. Because the TABP is an independent risk factor for coronary heart disease, it would be likely that behavioral hyperreactors are more common than silent ones; nonetheless the latter group could be a very significant demographic chunk.

We have attempted to establish a physiologic response underlying the TABP and link that response, by association, to coronary heart disease. Whether the pattern begets the physiology or vice versa is problematic, but it is likely that the two phenomena are intertwined, with the TABP a behavioral correlate of physiologic arousal in response to environmental stressors. Some researchers have speculated that the pattern evolved as a resource-gathering tool in competitive surroundings, and this does have conceptual appeal. It is, of course, possible that in this context the physiology evolved to support biologic requirements induced by the behavior, but this seems less sensible if we accept the premise that sympathomedullary arousal is a phylogenetically old mechanism long successful in aiding survival in a physically dangerous world, long predating complex aquisitive behaviors. To resolve this question, more information is needed as to the development of the behavior in children, any genetic basis for its occurrence (a most difficult subject to study in humans since it would almost seem to require separating children from parents to eliminate learned elements), the presence or absence of reactivity in larger populations of A and non-A children and adults, and perhaps studies in noncivilized populations as to the presence of reactivity and "A" attributes.

To explain observed sex differences in reactivity, one might theorize that a hunting–gathering existence such as that apparently led in early human cultures would generate greater cardiovascular arousal requirements in males who were the hunters than in female gatherers; that male competition for mates, resources, and shelter fostered the TABP; and that the two may have become genetically linked via the selection process. Regardless of the validity of such speculations, our civilized existence has modified the need for physiologic arousal and its behavioral concomitants.

Perhaps the evolutionary origins of the behavior are primarily of historical interest, but the developmental progress of the pattern in each generation is of vital clinical concern. If the behavior begins, as Butensky[28] suggests, as a situation-specific response in children, and progresses to a fixed trait whose physiologic correlates are present even under general anesthesia in later adulthood, than clearly a search must be instituted for ways to detect and modify deleterious aspects of the phenomena before they exert pathologic effects on the cardiovascular system. From our previous discussion, we can recall that in women the phenomena of both Type A behavior and hyperreactivity increase with age, and perhaps level of education. If our educational and employment priorities favor progressive development of this pattern, we may be wreaking significant epidemiologic havoc. However, as we stated at the end of the last chapter, it is not clear that all elements of the behavior are deleterious in terms of risk, and meager evidence from this chapter again demonstrates hostility and competitiveness as characteristics with apparently greater detrimental impact than other components of the pattern.

Most of the studies quoted in this chapter shared a common finding not previously mentioned. Type A individuals, or Type B individuals with CHD who were shown to be hyperreactive in response to a laboratory stressor, in every instance performed no better than their non-CHD Type B counterparts on the challenges set before them. The pattern and its physiology conferred no apparent advantage on those possessing it.

One criticism of all of these studies is the fact that the experimental challenges are contrived, and may have no relevance to real-life situations. We saw in the last chapter that the TABP may confer some scholastic advantage in college and in professional achievement. Certainly sympathomedullary arousal in certain circumstances of physical challenge can be lifesaving. A knowledge gasp between real-life and laboratory phenomena exists here, and for this reason my colleagues and I are striving to find ways to assess reactivity in day-to-day life.

Nonetheless the real-life analogs of laboratory situations are plentiful, and Type A's hyperresponsiveness to fundamentally trivial challenges is plain. In the next chapter, we dramatize the effects of "catecholamine storm" on the heart and vasculature, and make clear why sympathomedullary arousal to challenge is to be avoided unless true physical challenge is confronted, particularly in view of the fact that capacity to function under psychocognitive stress does not appear to be enhanced by such arousal. The disease entity of hypertension and its relationship to sympathetic arousal will be probed as well.

REFERENCES

1. Freidman, M., St. George, S., et al. Excretion of catecholamines, 17-ketosteroids, 17 hydroxycorticoids and 5-hydroxyindole in men exhibiting a particular behavior pattern (A) associated with high incidence of clinical coronary artery disease. *J Clin Inves*, 39:758–764, 1960.
2. Elmadjian, F., Hope, J. M., and Lamson, E. T. Excretion of epinephrine and norepinephrine under stress. *Rec Prog Horm Res*, 14:513, 1958.
3. Von Euler, U. S., Gemzell, C. A., et al. Cortical and medullary adrenal activity in emotional stress. *Acta Endocr (Kbh)*, 30:567, 1959.
4. Freidman, M., Byers, S. O., et al. Plasma catecholamine response of coronary-prone subjects (Type A) to a specific challenge. *Metabolism*, 24:205–210, 1975.
5. Stern, R. M., Ray, W. J., and Davis, C. M. *Psychophysiological recording*. New York: Oxford University Press, 1980.
6. Manuck, S. B., Craft, S., and Gold, K. J. Coronary-prone behavior pattern and cardiovascular response. *Psychophysiology*, 15:403–411, 1978.
7. Dembrowski, T. M., MacDougall, J. M., et al. Components of the Type A coronary-prone behavior pattern and cardiovascular response to psychomotor performance challenge. *J Behav Med*, 1:159–176, 1978.
8. Dembrowski, T. M., MacDougall, J. M., and Lushene, R. Interpersonal interaction and cardiovascular response in Type A subjects and coronary patients. *J Hum Stress*, 5:28–36, 1979.
9. Dembrowski, T. M., MacDougasll, J. M., et al. Effect of level of challenge on pressor and heart rate responses in Type A and B subjects. *J Appl Soc Psychol*, 9:209–228, 1979.
10. Goldband, S. Stimulus specificity of physiological response to stress and the Type A coronary-prone behavior pattern. *J Pers Soc Psychol*, 39:670–679, 1980.
11. Obrist, P. A., Light, K. C., et al. Behavior research methods and instrumentation, *Psychophysiology*, 10:623–626, 1978.
12. Keys, A., Taylor, H. L., et al. Mortality and coronary heart disease among men studied for 23 years. *Arch Intern Med*, 128:201–214, 1971.

13. Gastorf, J. W. Physiologic reaction of Type A's to objective and subjective challenge. *J Hum Stress*, 7:16–20, 1981.
14. Pittner, M. S., and Houston, B. K. Response to stress, cognitive coping strategies, and the Type A behavior pattern. *J Pers Soc Psychol*, 39:147–157, 1980.
15. Blumenthal, J. A., Lane, J. D., et al. Effect of task incentive on cardiovascular response in Type A and Type B individuals. *Psychophysiology*, 20:63–69, 1983.
16. Manuck, S. B., and Garland, F. N. Coronary-prone behavior pattern, task incentive, and cardiovascular response. *Psychophysiology*, 16:136–142, 1979.
17. Schwartzx, P. J., and Weiss, T. T-wave amplitude as an index of cardiac sympathetic activity: A misleading concept. *Psychophysiology*, 20:696–702, 1983.
18. Heslegrave, R. L., and Furedy, J. J. On the utility of T-wave amplitude: A reply to Schwartz and Weiss. *Psychophysiology*, 20:702–709, 1983.
19. Lane, J. D., White, A. D., et al. Cardiovascular effects of mental arithmetic in Type A and Type B females. *Psychophysiology*, 21:39–46, 1984.
20. MacDougall, J. M., Dembrowski, T. M., and Krantz, D. S. Effects of types of challenge on pressor and heart rate responses in Type A and B women. *Psychophysiology*, 18:1–9, 1981.
21. Aslan, S., Nelson, L., et al. Stress and age effects on catecholamines in normal subjects. *J Psychosom Res*, 25:33–41, 1981.
22. Frankenhauser, M., Wright, M. R. V., et al. Sex differences in psychoendocrine reactions to examination stress. *Psychosom Med*, 40:334–339, 1978.
23. Collins, M., and Frankenhauser, M. Stress responses in male and female engineering students. *J Hum Stress*, 4:43–47, 1978.
24. Waldron, I., Zyzanski, S., et al. The coronary-prone behavior pattern in employed men and women. *J Hum Stress*, 3:2–18, 1977.
25. Waldron, I. The coronary-prone behavior pattern, blood pressure, employment, and socioeconomic status in women. *J Psychosom Res*, 22:79–87, 1978.
26. Lawler, K. A., Rixse, A., and Allen, M. T. Type AS behavior and psychophysiologic responses in adult women. *Psychophysiology*, 20:343–350, 1983.
27. Matthews, K. A., and Angulo, J. Measurement of the Type A behavior pattern in children: Assessment of children's competitiveness, Impatience-anger, and aggression. *Child Dev*, 51:466–475, 1980.
28. Butensky, A., Faralli, V., et al. Elements of the coronary-prone behavior pattern in children and teen-agers. *J Psychosom Res*, 20:439–444, 1976.
29. Lundberg, U. Note on type A behavior and cardiovascular responses to challenge in 3-6 year old children. *J Psychosom Res*, 27:39–42, 1983.
30. Lawler, K. A., Allen, M. T., et al. The relationship of physiological responses to the coronary-prone behavior pattern in children. *J Behav Med*, 4:203–216, 1981.
31. Kahn, J. P., Kornfeld, D. S., et al. Type A behavior and blood pressure during coronary bypass surgery. *Psychosom Med*, 42:407–414, 1980.
32. Krantz, D. S., Arabian, J. M., et al. Type A behavior and coronary artery bypass surgery: Intraoperative blood pressure and perioperative complications. *Psychosom Med*, 44:273–284, 1982.

33. Corse, C. D., Manuck, S. B., et al. Coronary-prone behavior pattern and cardiovascular response in persons with and without coronary heart disease. *Psychosom Med*, 44:449–459, 1982.
34. Sime, W. E., Buell, J. C., et al. Electrocardiogram and blood pressure responses to emotional stress (quiz interview) in post-infarct cardiac patients and matched control subjects. *J Hum Stress*, 6:39–46, 1980.
35. Simpson, M., Oleivine, D., et al. Exercise-induced catecholamines and platelet-aggregation in the cornoary-prone behavior pattern. *Psychosom Med*, 36:476–487, 1974.

5

THE GATHERING CLOUDS: TENSION, HYPERTENSION, AND TYPE A BEHAVIOR

Why are some of us Type A? Being "A" is no more effective in terms of performance in the laboratory situation, but it may well be on the battlefield, in the acquisition of food and shelter, and perhaps in the corporate and academic worlds, as well. Some[1] have speculated that it evolved as a means of controlling one's environment. Others[2] feel it is a vestigial remnant of early resource-acquiring behavior. Perhaps the two are not very different; one can easily envision an animal that is more aggressive, hostile, competitive, and ambitious and is hyperalert as being more successful in a world that seems to select for such characteristics when resources are limited. In today's "civilized" world of largely nonphysical interaction, however, are potential benefits of the behavior worth the cost? In Chapter 3 we alluded to the fact that in academic circles, at least, the behavior pattern may well accrue some benefits. We must judge this for ourselves, but the toll must be understood if one is to choose wisely and consciously rather than be a victim of behavioral patterns that appear to have evolved to cope with a far more hostile environment than that we now endure. Further, when we approach a Type A patient from a therapeutic perspective, we must be able to aid that individual in understanding how his or her perceptions of the environment and subsequent behavior might impact the patient's present and future health.

THE GATHERING CLOUDS

What we must do is to propose a way in which behavioral responses might contribute to the pathogenesis, or causality, of the disease in question.

If we are to invoke any mechanism in the pathogenesis of coronary heart disease, it will be useful to review briefly just what we currently believe to be the actual processes causing the occlusions in coronary arteries. The anatomic lesions of CHD are well described; they consist of plugs of cholesterol, calcium, clotted blood, and fibrous or scar tissue that progressively narrow the lumen of the artery and restrict blood flow. These "plaques" appear to begin as proliferation of the muscle cells lining the vessel wall, perhaps in response to chronic injury, with cholesterol and other fats becoming deposited within these cells. From this point, fats seem to be deposited *between* the cells, followed by fibrous tissue. Hemorrhage (or bleeding) and calcium deposits ensue, progressively plugging the vessel, and rendering the lesion apparently irreversible. Clotting elements in the bloodstream, known as platelets, appear to play a role by becoming deposited on the rough surfaces of the plaque and initiating further clot formation (Figure 7).

Exactly what initiates the original cellular proliferation remains a mystery, but vascular wear-and-tear from episodic or sustained hypertension is a leading contender. This wear-and-tear initiates a healing–scarring process that results in plaque formation.

Another theory advanced in recent years is that the vessel wall sustains minor nonspecific injury over time, thus presenting a very slightly roughened surface to the stream of blood. Platelets, elements in the blood that are designed to respond to injury, adhere to the wall, instigating clot formation and the rest of the afore-described events. Here the initiating event is not extraordinary; under normal circumstances platelets bypass minor injury, but, for some reason, in patients prone to coronary disease, the platelets are abnormally sticky.

According to the one theory, the basic pathology lies in a response to excessive injury; the other purports an excessive response to minimal injury.[3]

Irrespective of the initiating event, it appears virtually certain that each of the identifiable risk factors discussed in Chapter 3 must exert its influence at some stage in this process, probably quite early. What must also be kept in mind is that the risk factors appears to operate *independently*, and the more risk factors one possesses, the more likelyhood there is of developing the disease. Therefore, we cannot ascribe the impact of the Type A pattern on coronary disease as a function, say, of an increased incidence of cigarette abuse within this population. There may well be interactions between the risk factors, as we shall discuss, but we must search for contributions to causality within each risk factor.

We have thus far demonstrated the association between the Type A behavior pattern (TABP) and coronary heart disease, cardiovascular hyperreactivity and TABP, and possibly reactivity and coronary disease, independent of behavioral typology. We speculated that there may exist so-called "silent reactors" who do not display the outward manifestations of reactivity—namely, the Type A pattern—but who become physiologically aroused in the face of cognitive or emotional challenge. Coronary disease is seen to be more common in these individuals than in matched controls. This would

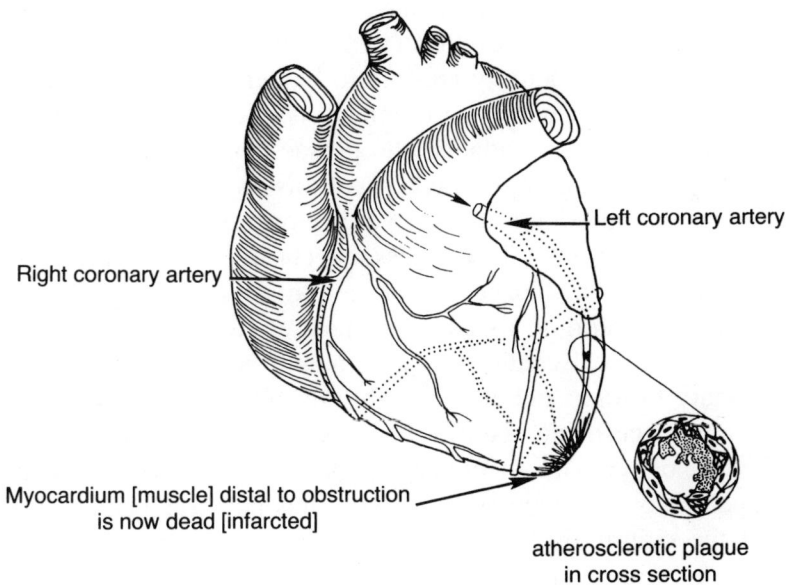

Figure 7.

all seem to suggest that cardiovascular hyperreactivity may be a link between psychogenic stress and coronary heart disease. If reactivity is an expression of sympathomedullary arousal, as we have shown is probably the case, then it would seem that arousal itself is a final common pathway between stress and disease. This chapter will explore that premise, which does appear intuitively sensible.

Sympathomedullary arousal is a well-described stress response, discussed at length in Chapter 2. Let us review it briefly. Arousal, stimulated by threat or challenge, occurs as a consequence of the outpouring of impulses from the brain to the sympathetic nervous system and to the adrenal medulla, resulting in the release of epinephrine from the latter and norepinephrine from nerve terminals of the former. This results in a rather stereotypic pattern of physiologic and biochemical alterations, including an increase in the rate and force of cardiac contraction; a redistribution of blood flow to skeletal musculature, heart, and brain and away from the skin and gastrointestinal tract; elevation of the blood pressure; dilation of the airways and pupils; and various metabolic alterations apparently designed to make energy-yielding substrates available to the stressed organism.

Such homeostatic alterations have value when abrupt, vigorous activity is called for, and have been termed fight-or-flight responses. Subsequent physical activity appears to be performed with greater alacrity and strength when the organism is under the influence of the catecholamines. Individuals who pursue dangerous sports such as mountain climbing or sky diving call this an "adrenaline rush" and describe an alteration in their perceptions of the environment, which assume a prenatural sharpness and clarity, and in which time seems to slow down. Indeed, many seek this experience as a thrill or "high," proclaiming its addictive nature. Repetitive arousal in response to physical challenge was probably a way of life in our evolutionary history, and also probably of great adaptive value.

The more germane issue now, however, is what the consequences are of sympathomedullary arousal when elicited frequently and repetitively by challenge *not* requiring physical response. Is arousal the culprit that links the Type A pattern, and other hot reactors, to coronary disease? This will occupy us for the remainder of this chapter, and the next as well. We explore the consequences of reactivity, to ascertain if and where the link occurs.

THE GATHERING CLOUDS

We begin with blood pressure elevation in response to catecholamines, or the phenomenon of hypertension.

In the following chapter, our inquiry involves alterations in blood pressure, alterations in cardiac electrical activity, direct damage to the heart muscle from catecholamines, and consequences of the metabolic alterations during arousal. We explore how catecholamines might effect platelet stickiness and fat deposition in cells, as well. We will than be able to reconsider the question asked earlier: Is it worth it?

Elevations in blood pressure, as mentioned earlier, might result in vascular injury over time, the so-called wear-and-tear hypothesis. We now investigate whether sympathomedullary arousal can result in sustained hypertension, a risk factor clearly shown to contribute to coronary disease, probably by this mechanism.

Because so many individuals are hypertensive in their own right, a thorough understanding of the association between this disorder and stress would be most helpful.

A rather fascinating initial observation is that it has been shown repeatedly that Type A individuals are *not* more likely to be chronically hypertensive than B's. Many of the studies in the last chapter documented no blood-pressure differences at rest between the two groups, and epidemiologic research has failed to uncover an increased incidence in A's of the disease entity known as essential hypertension. We have also emphasized repeatedly the independent nature of risk factors. Hence we must leave Type A's behind for this portion of the investigation, and look at the relationship between sympathomedullary arousal and essential hypertension, not the episodic bursts seen in A's in response to challenge. We must postulate other mechanisms for the A–coronary disease link.

Essential hypertension is an enigma to both clinicians and researchers. The very name signifies that we have essentially no idea what causes it. However, it long has been suspected that there is a link between brain and body in the pathogenesis of the process (again note "hyper-tension") but this has yet to be proved definitively, at least to the satisfaction of writers of most scholarly texts and reviews of the subject. The reader will again be asked to judge as we proceed to explore this link. This judgment may have profound impact on an attitudes towards the care of patients with this disease.

The term hypertension is now taken to mean an elevation of the blood pressure in the arteries of the body. This can occur as a result of an excessive volume of fluid in the vessels (overfilling the pipes), an increase in the resistance of the blood vessels to the movement of blood (narrowing the pipes), or an increase in the output of the heart (turning up the pump). It is felt that there are elements of each operating in individuals with essential hypertension. Our primary interest is how sympathomedullary arousal might contribute to any of these processes.

Each of these three mechanisms could easily be influenced by sympathetic arousal. Recall that sympathetic arousal is triggered in the face of physical challenge or injury, and has the adaptive function of enabling the body to perform beyond normal capability or to respond to a sudden decrease in blood pressure caused by bleeding (shock). An increase in cardiac output, as we already know, is a primary and important consequence of sympathetic activation, as is constriction of blood vessels, especially to nonexercising tissue. The third possible mechanism for increased blood pressure, overfilling the pipes, might occur as a result of excessive salt and water being held in the blood vessels by the kidney. Besides the red blood cells, these are the primary components of blood.

In fact, the kidney does have a mechanism to do just that, so that in the face of bleeding or dehydration urine production diminishes and blood volume is conserved. This is mediated via the hormone renin, released by the kidney when sensors in this organ detect low blood pressure. The triggering mechanism for this cascade is a diminution of blood flow to the kidney, caused by constriction of its feeder artieries, and mediated by sympathetic nervous activation. This, of course, meshes nicely with the rest of the stress response by conserving blood for exercising or, more immediately, vital organs, and at the same time conserving body fluids.

(Note that there other causes for hypertension besides that termed essential, such as kidney failure and certain types of tumors, but these are rare and need not concern us here.)

Like most other diseases, essential hypertension has to start somewhere, and some of the most interesting and enlightening studies relevant to arousal have been done in young, so-called "prehypertensives," also termed "borderline" or "labile" hypertensive individuals. These individuals, often with a family history of essential hypertension, have episodic, abnormal elevations in their blood pressure, frequently in response to stressful stimuli. Such individuals have been shown frequently to progress to the fixed hypertensive state.[4-6] Many of these studies follow formats familiar to us from the last chapter, where groups of (in this case) labile or normotensive adolescents or college students are subjected to various laboratory stressors—physical, cognitive, or emotional—and their physiological and biochemical responses measured. Notably absent are attempts to induce competition or to threaten ego; in other words, to provoke Type A behavior specifically. Several of the studies separate patients based only on the presence or absence of essential hypertension in the parent, predicated on the assumption that family history constitutes a prehypertensive state.[1,6,7]

In general, their results demonstrate that both labile hypertensives (normotensive with occasionally elevated casual readings) and family-history-positive individuals react more intensely physiologically to a variety of psychogenic stressors with elevations of both blood pressure and heart rate despite baselines similar to those of the controls.[1,2,4,6-11] Sounds familiar? Also familiar is the fact that not all studies concur. However, out of the number reviewed, only one differed to an appreciable extent, and I was unable to find any definition of how their labile hypertensives were differentiated from normotensives.[11] Sample size was small (total of 15), as well.

A few of these studies deserve a closer look. One[10] demonstrated a hierarchy of responsiveness with labile hypertensive adolescents with a positive family history the most reactive, followed by normotensives with a positive family history, with both responses significantly different from those of controls. In addition, poststress catecholamines followed the same pattern, with positive family history labile hypertensives having the highest values. A potentially important finding that will occupy us more fully later was the persistence of elevations in blood pressure in the labile group and some of the normotensive positive-family-history individuals after the test, despite normal baselines.

Once again, we see a population of hyperresponsive individuals who appear to undergo sympathomedullary arousal in response to stressors. In looking more closely, we can again define certain circumstances that appear to be more potent in eliciting that arousal than others, circumstances different from what arouses Type A's. Two studies specifically address this issue: both compare the capability of active tasks, such as video games versus passive stressors such as sticking one's arm in a bucket of cold water or watching a disturbing movie to elicit cardiovascular reactivity. Active stressors in both cases were the most potent in eliciting arousal. There was no association in either research between Type A behavior and reactivity, however, no attempt was made to provoke the pattern in that the tests were blandly administered without competitive or challenging overtones.

It appears that we are defining two distinct populations of hyperreactors that do not seem to overlap: the TABP individual hyperresponsive to TABP-relevant challenges, and the labile hypertensive reactive to active coping tasks that are not designed to elicit A behaviors. Most work fails to demonstrate any association between the TABP, labile, or positive-family-history hypertension and cardiovascular reactivity to non-A-provoking stressors.[9,25,31] Both states appear to place the patient at risk for the development of coronary disease, and both states appear to be associated with sympathomedullary arousal to psychogenic stressors. Yet the pathologic pathways seem to diverge at this point, with the apparent mechanism of coronary risk in prehypertensives the development of hypertension, and in TABP individuals no fixed hypertension, but some other consequence of the arousal as yet unelucidated.

One might argue that sympathomedullary arousal to stressors has little to do with the development of essential hypertension; perhaps they are both part of the same underlying abnormality, and are an association rather than a cause. Certainly the failure of medical teaching to emphasize stress responses as pathogenic mechanisms for the development of hypertension would seem to imply that this is the case. But let us examine it more closely. If we could show that episodic responsiveness in certain predisposed individuals could lead to a fixed hypertensive state, then it would follow that essential hypertension is *preventable*, by blunting responsiveness either behaviorally or pharmacologically. If we could show a similar phenomenon in Type A's, then it might be possible to decrease the incidence of coronary heart disease by dealing effectively with the mechanisms behind the risk factor.

An intriguing and somewhat disturbing fact is that medical literature exists that would support such a premise. Let us look first at prehypertensives and hypertensives and examine the role of sympathomedullary arousal in the causality of such states. We have already demonstrated the presence of increased catecholamines in response to challenge in labile hypertensives,[10,12,14] although this is not universal.[11] (Note that we are not discussing the reactivity or catecholamine responses of patients with fixed, essential hypertension.) Does such sympathomedullary arousal create or contribute to the development of essential hypertension? We have already noted that labile hypertension appears epidemiologically to be a precursor to development of this disease, as does the presence of a family history of the illness. Is inappropriate, episodic arousal the link?

We can look to animal studies where genetically borderline hypertensive rats were rendered persistently and profoundly hypertensive by conflict situations in which they were punished unpredictably for their responses to stimuli.[15] The same researchers[16] demonstrated severe cardiac abnormalities in these rats, consisting of inflammation, muscle scarring, and tissue breakdown. No mention is made of the coronary arteries, however. The authors of these studies feel there are certain analogies between their model of genetically predisposed rats developing fixed hypertension in response to stressors and human labile hypertensives. The sustained hypertension, however, was studied for only ten weeks, and a similarly designed study[18] demonstrated the return of blood pressure to normal in most of its subjects after 13 weeks of no stress. (Note that the rat strains were not the same.) Generally, animal researchers have had great difficulty in creating hypertension in rats in response to most stressors.[15]

This, of course, tells us more about rats than about people, and animal models of psychogenic stress are difficult to analogize with the human condition. Human prehypertensives are more reactive to certain stressors, and are more prone to become hypertensive. One might now ask: Are fixed hypertensives more hyperreactive?

Certain studies suggest that this is so. In the usual format, these patients have been compared with normotensive or both normotensive and "labotensive" populations in terms of their responses to various stressors.[8,18-23] All of these studies were able to demonstrate an increased reactivity of hypertensives, with labiles being intermediate when this group was included. The agreement is not universal, however, and there are almost as many data demonstrating no differences[11,20,24-27] or even hyporeactivity among established

THE GATHERING CLOUDS

hypertensives.[36] Steptoe[8] in the most recent study of this subject to date, discusses these differences. He points out that there are at least three confounding variables in the way these studies are performed that might profoundly influence the results.

1. Patient selection. Mixed groups of patients with different severities of hypertension and different treatment regimens have been used. Both of these, as we shall discuss, may dramatically alter physiologic responsiveness.

2. The recruitment of patients and normal controls. The stated diagnosis of hypertension to someone who has not previously been told he or she has the disease may influence subsequent perceptions of stressful events. On the other hand, normal controls, who are often recruited from the laboratory or hospital environs, may be much more comfortable in the experimental situation than a patient to whom the experience is novel, and it is clear that the novelty of a stressor is important in delimiting the stress response.

3. Variable nature of stressors. A problem addressed previously, it can be invoked readily to explain variable results.

It is worthwhile to look more closely at some of these studies, because despite the conflicting data and confounding variables, coherence is on the horizon.

It has been hypothesized that the disease of essential hypertension passes through stages in its progression from the labile state. That progression may occur both physiologically and psychologically, and may explain the variance in the data on the reactivity of the fixed hypertensive. With reference to our earlier discussion of the pathogenesis of the disease, we commented that it was probably due to various combinations of increased intravascular volume, increased resistance to blood flow, and increased output of the heart. It has been hypothesized that the initial stages of hypertension rely more on an increased output in the heart, possibly in response to catecholamines, and, over time, chronic changes in the blood vessels, with progressive narrowing in response to the continued pressure overload.[28] The output of the heart then diminishes in an attempt to maintain homeostasis, and the hypertension becomes based primarily on the increased vascular resistance.[29]

That is not the whole story. Hyperreactivity, it appears, does not operate so selectively in these prehypertensive individuals, but involves the vasculature as well as the heart. A noninvasive[20] and an invasive[24] study—with the latter involving catheterization of arteries, which allows more effective calculation of vascular resistance—both showed an increase in vascular resistance from constriction of blood vessels in response to anxiety-provoking situations in normotensive and hypertensive individuals. Both studies involved relatively young patients (oldest 45) and similar stressors. The results were parallel, and afford some clues as to the mechanism of reactivity. In both studies hypertensives and normotensive controls increased their blood pressures and their vascular resistances in response to the stressors. The patterns were similar; the differences between the normotensives and hypertensives were quantitative rather than qualitative, and the authors conclude that the arousal seen in hypertensives is merely an exaggerated normal response to stress. The aroused state in these studies persisted longer in the hypertensives than in normals. However, it is still not quite that simple.

Two other studies suggest differences in the *patterns* of arousal between hypertensives and normotensives that have important implications.[21,23] Both showed a selective diminution of blood flow to the kidney in hypertensive individuals subjected to stress as compared with normals. The most recent of these studies found the difference "striking" and it occurred in response to a mild stressor designed not to provoke major arousal.[21] This "fools" the kidney into acting as if the organism is in shock because the diminished blood flow activates the low blood pressure sensors and causes release of the hormone renin. Salt and water are conserved, intravascular volume increases, and blood pressure rises. The hypertensive is reacting to a psychological stressor in such a fashion as to increase blood pressure. (Figure 8).

Individuals in that study with positive family histories showed similar abnormalities, although less pronounced. Animal studies[31] have demonstrated salt and water retention in response to stress, most marked in genetically hypertensive strains.[30] A human study in labile hypertensives[32] found that psychological stress induced salt and water retention in young men who were either labile hypertensives or had a family history as compared with low-risk controls. What was particularly notable about this work was that it was only

THE GATHERING CLOUDS

high heart rate reactors in response to stress that demonstrated this abnormality. All of these hot reactors were in the prehypertensive groups.

Note that this is more than a quantitative difference in response, such as we saw with vascular resistance. There is a clear difference in kidney blood flow changes in normals, on the one hand, and in hypertensives and prehypertensives, on the other. Many normals actually displayed an *increase* in kidney blood flow in response to stress.[21]

We have now managed to tie three pathogenic mechanisms of hypertension to the stress response: increased cardiac output, increased vascular resistance, and increased blood volume. We have seen each of these mechanisms at work in both the fixed hypertensive state and the preessential hypertensive. We have seen these mechanisms stimulated in both animals and humans in response to psychogenic stimuli.

Although much of this work has been reported in journals read primarily by clinical psychologists, research physiologists, or specialists in "psychosomatic medicine," the clinical medical literature

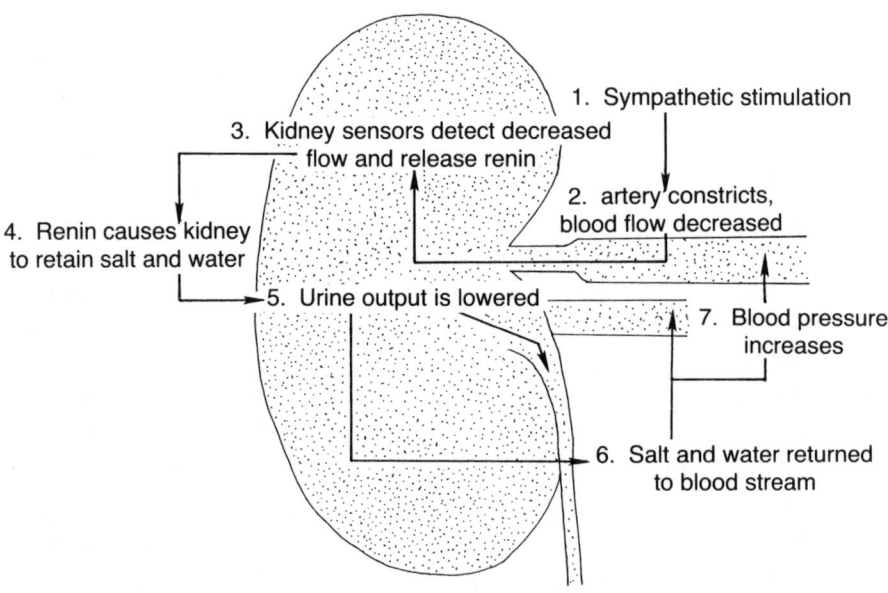

Figure 8.

has not been exempt. A study in the prestigious *New England Journal of Medicine* in 1977 documented a subpopulation of "mild essential hypertensives" who had baseline elevations in their blood renin.[33] This group was also found to have elevated blood catecholamine levels as compared with the normal renin group and a set of matched normotensive controls. A number of pharmacologic machinations of the sympathetic nervous system and renin secretion were undertaken, which demontrated that these elevated catecholamines were unrelated to the elevation of renin per se, and when blockade of the sympathetic nervous system was accomplished, this group displayed normal blood pressures, unlike the other (normal renin) hypertensives. (We discuss this blockade more extensively in the next chapter.) The implication is that these hypertensives are so probably because their renin levels are elevated as a result of chronic, low-grade arousal. One might not be surprised to learn that this group displayed an excess of "suppressed hostility" on psychological testing. The conclusions of these researchers are worth quoting:

> We have attempted to delineate a subset of patients with mild essential hypertension in whom plasma renin activity is elevated, and sympathetic nervous activity is increased, the hypertension appears to be neurogenic (i.e., originating in the nervous system) and psychosomatic mechanisms may be important . . . to what extent, if at all, hypertension in these patients progresses to moderate and severe grades is uncertain. The fact that plasma renin activity is normal or low in the majority of patients with established or essential hypertension, older patients, or those with moderately severe disease, does not exclude the possibility of such a progression, since plasma renin activity and sympathetic nervous responsiveness in essential hypertension fall with aging and increasing severity of the hypertensive process. [statements referenced]

Perhaps here lies the key that might explain the discrepancies in cardiovascular reactivity in individuals with established hypertension. It may be that their location in the progression of disease will determine their reactivity. It has been suggested[18] that the increase in vascular tone becomes fixed as a result of actual structural alerations in the vessels themselves, and there is, therefore, a diminished capacity to respond to arousal. Perhaps blood pressure "homeostats" eventually become resent at higher levels after repeated elevations in response to everyday events. As one researcher commented: "There is no evidence that patients with essential hypertension are more exposed to pain, cold, waiting, examinations or arithmetic tests, than normotensives. But there is evidence that such patients live in or experience their life situations as more stressful than normatensives."[24]

Furthermore, it has been demonstrated in experimental animals that situational blood pressure elevations may cause changes in the blood pressure of the kidney over time—an event that may alter water and salt handling and the level of blood pressure.[34,35] Certainly it is clear that in humans long-standing hypertension causes significant damage to kidneys, and may ultimately be the cause of demise in this disease.

These chronic vascular changes occurring in long-standing hypertension might explain why not all essential hypertensives are found to be hyperreactors to stressful stimuli; their vesels are no longer capable of such responses. Perhaps, though, there is another dimension that involves how the long-term hypertensive perceives stress and so reacts to it. Perhaps in addition to the structural alterations, the hypertensive's perceptions of stimuli evolve as well, with diminished reactivity the result. Let us investigate this interesting possibility.

Some data exist in support of this premise. Hypertensive individuals have been characterized as "insulated" and "distant" by a group of researchers who attempted to stimulate emotions and measure responsiveness to fantasies projected onto images presented on cards designed for this purpose. Military personnel were asked to tell a story evoked by these images when shown the cards. (*Content* of the fantasy was found to be largely irrelevant to the concomitant physiologic response.) Individuals with established hypertension were found to be *hypo*reactive, to be far more concrete and literal in their stories, and to display little emotional involvement. They interacted minimally with the experimenter during the procedure, which correlated with a lack of physiologic reactivity on the part of these individuals as compared with nonhypertensive controls.[36] An older study involving psychodrama drew similar conclusions.[37]

A third study[22] investigated perceptual differences between hypertensive and normotensive patients by showing both groups two movies depicting two types of doctor–patient interactions. One physician appeared rude and disinterested, and the other warm and caring. The experimenters had thought that the "bad" doctor would serve as a stressor and elicit a hypertensive response; this did not occur, to their initial disappointment. What they noted, instead, was a failure of the hypertensive group to differentiate the two physicians according to their behavior, or at least a failure to verbalize this perception. A few of the hypertensives actually switched the two, referring quite specifically to the "bad" doctor as "good." More frequently, hypertensives indicated no difference between the physicians.

Upon reading partial transcripts of the interviews provided with the paper, I personally was impressed by the literal nature of the hypertensive's perceptions of the differences between the two physicians, for instance, "one took the pressure in both arms" and "one took his glasses off." The role differences between the two physicians were far from subtle. I was truly struck by the apparent failure of the hypertensives to perceive this.

The theory advanced by these researchers is that the hypertensive individual may "screen out potentially noxious stimuli as a defense against his cardiovascular reactivity." This implies a below-consciousness learning process that effectively screens out those perceptions that might enhance reactivity. The process does not appear to occur on a cognitive level. One is reminded of a generic failure of some individuals to "see the writing on the wall"; that is, to deny the existence of the unpleasant because of the uncomfortable feelings evoked.

On the basis of these data, it would seem to be worthwhile to explore more broadly the emotional structure of the hypertensive.

Literature exists that examines the hypertensive in this light. While the Type A is characterized as aggressive, ambitious, and hostile, some researchers claim that the hypertensive withholds expressions of emotion, particularly anger, a trait known as "anger-in." This has been the subject of several studies,[33,38–44] two of which we review here.

The first is a study, discussed previously,[33] that demonstrates a subset of hypertensive patients characterized by high renin levels who were cardiovascular hyperreactors. This study also found that the high-renin hypertensives exhibited "marked" differences from low-renin hypertensives according to various measures of suppressed hostility. In addition, the authors state: "The overall personality profile was one of controlled, guilt-prone, submissive persons with a high level of unexpressed anger."

A series of studies[40-44] reported by one investigative team over the past ten years addressed specifically the anger-in coping style as a predictor of hypertensive disease. The studies were carried out in two distinct socioeconomic settings, one termed high stress and the other termed low stress on the basis of crime rates, divorce incidence, median income and education, and percent unemployment. A total of just over 1000 subjects—black and white, male and female—were surveyed for the presence of hypertension, and requested to complete a questionnaire that asked for their responses to five "provocative interpersonal situations." The situations involved hypothetical unprovoked aggression by a spouse, police officer, landlord, or other individual, and respondents were classified as anger-in or anger-out, depending upon their willingness to "show" their feelings. The results of the series can be summarized as follows:

1. Black and white males in both socio-economic settings who displayed anger-in coping had significantly higher diastolic blood pressures and greater incidence of hypertensive disease than anger-out individuals.

2. Black females in high-stress areas and white females in low-stress areas were also more likely to be hypertensive if they were "anger-in copers," but not white high-stress or black low-stress residents.

3. A recent comprehensive look at the pooled data demonstrated that being black, female, living in a high-stress area, and coping with a variety of situations with "anger-in" were all potent risk factors for being hypertensive.

A study on a much smaller scale that specifically addressed the anger issue demonstrated elevated catecholamine levels in hypertensives associated with a much higher (53 versus 18) percentage of these individuals displaying anger-in traits on a self-questionnaire.[27]

These ideas are not new. In 1939 Alexander[45] suggested that chronic anger inhibition results eventually in hypertensive disease. It is sometimes difficult for mechanistic thinkers such as physicians to accept the validity of behavior data. To put these findings into perspective, however, we need a few additional facts. It has been demonstrated[38,39,46] that anger elevates blood pressure. It has been further demonstrated[46-48] that this is accomplished via sympathetic nervous activation and, as expected, is accompanied by elevated catecholamine levels. Finally, if the anger has no outlet, the hypertensive response is greater than if openly expressed.[38,39]

A picture of certain hypertensives begins to emerge. An individual, frequently with a family history of hypertensive disease, tends to display sympathomedullary arousal to the stressors of daily life. This arousal results in episodic elevations in both cardiac output and vascular resistance, increases in blood renin levels, and resulting abnormal salt and water retention. When exposed to stressors capable of arousing even normotensives, the reactivity tends to be of greater degree, and to persist longer. Over time pathologic changes occur, very likely in the blood vessel walls and probably in the kidney, such that the blood pressure elevation converts from an episodic to a fixed condition. Stressors no longer have the capacity to elicit further elevations in pressure, as the system becomes less dynamic in response to the pathologic changes. Emotionally, one might hypothesize, the patient has long been internalizing feelings, particularly anger and hostility. Over time the patient becomes insulated and distant, with perceptions of life events being altered to achieve those states.

What we have done is to create a model of hypertension to fit the observed data from the studies we have discussed. The weak points of the model are that insufficient data are available to be able to characterize most, or even many, hypertensives as insulated, etc. The evolutionary course is purely hypothetical, and the major missing link is a longitudinal long-term study that follows the physiologic and behavioral changes of prehypertensives over many years. Demographically we know that many of these individuals will go on to become fixed hypertensives, but perceptual alterations accompanying this transition, as well as the details of the physiologic changes, are only surmised.

This does not invalidate the model. Most of the contradictions in the cited studies are defensible on the grounds of differing severity (and hence evolutionary level) of the hypertensive state, the presence or absence of treatment (a major confounding factor because most of such treatments blunt sympathetic arousal), and differences in experimental design. The psychological studies are in rather astounding agreement on the emotional characteristics of at least certain groups of hypertensives. I personally am willing to accept this model at least as a working clinical tool, and as a step toward an understanding of the stressor–stress response interaction in creating disease. Hypertension in its own right is a significant cause of morbidity and mortality, and its interface with coronary disease is demographically unquestioned, if poorly understood metchanistically.

One thing that is apparent from the model is that labile hypertensives are quite different in their psychological profiles than Type A's, even though they share sympathomedullary response to stressors. Two questions still need to be addressed in this regard: (1) Are the stressors to which they respond the same? (2) Are the *patterns* of physiologic response the same?

We can address the first question initially by noting that studies on the TABP have tended to employ stressors whose content is designed to be relevant to the Type A construct, whereas such studies in labile and fixed hypertensives have generally made no attempt to do this. Specifically, competition, time urgency, and threat to self-esteem are the most potent in eliciting "A" reactivity. These dimensions were not stressed in most of the challenges presented to labile hypertensives. We have noted the inability of those challenges to stimulate A's, and one might infer that the stresses were not adequate to elicit arousal[4-8] or the arousal was undetected by the usual measures. This is a possibility we will elaborate on shortly.

Actually, a group has studied A's in the context of stressors very much like those discussed in the hypertension reactivity papers referred to in this chapter. Forced mental arithmetic, word association, and digit substitution tasks given without competitive instructions failed to result in "A" hyperreactivity across a variety of physiologic measures. Indeed B's were more reactive according to some of the parameters measured[49] We spent a good deal of time in the last chapter detailing what makes A's react. We see now that a variety of challenges can be presented to A's that do not appeaer to induce them to become physiologically aroused, tasks that can arouse other populations—the labile hypertensives.

The second question, regarding patterns of response, is rather critical. We know both groups are hyperreactors, though perhaps to different stimuli. However, is the stress response stereotypic and identical? We have seen, in general, elevations of blood pressure, and frequently of heart rate, in response to their particular stressors in both groups. Some studies have utilized other measures, including direct measurements of cardiac output and indirect measures of vascular resistance. Others have measured catecholamines concomitantly. We know that at least certain hypertensives demonstrate differences in kidney blood flow from normals and other hypertensives. This suggests that not all patterns of arousal are the same.

It has been suggested that there occur three relatively distinct patterns of cardiovascular reactivity.[50] These have been termed (1) hypertonic if they are predominantly vasoconstrictive in nature, noted clinically by an elevated systolic and diastolic blood pressure and cold, clammy extremities—essentially a state of increased vascular resistance; (2) hyperkinetic, analogous to the physiologic response to exercise, with rapid heart rate, increased blood flow to skeletal muscle, increased systolic and *decreased* diastolic pressure (termed increased pulse pressure and measured by subtracting diastolic from systolic blood pressure, all of which constitute a high-output, decreased resistance state; and (3) mixed reactivity, with elements of both, probably including elevated renin levels (Figure 9).[11]

We have already noted that, at least initially, labile hypertensives display a mixed pattern that may progress to predominantly hypertonic or vasoconstrictive. The hyperkinetic response makes imminent sense to a fighting or fleeing organism, which will require much blood delivered to the working muscles of the body. Groen et al.[24] propose that the hyperkinetic phase may give rise to the hypertonic pattern if the physiologic arousal is not converted into muscular activity because of behavioral inhibitions (i.e., refraining from hitting the boss despite the boss's intransigence). They feel that this is what facilitates the development of chronic essential (vasoconstrictive) hypertension, an interesting corollary to the "anger-in" concept.

There is a recent article that purports to demonstrate a more predominantly hyperkinetic response of A's to challenge that was not accompanied by harassment. What was demonstrated was an increase in plasma catecholamines to forced mental arithmetic in A's accompanied by an increase in flow to skeletal muscle without any differences in blood pressure or heart rate.[51] This suggests that reactivity in A's may well have been present in other studies, but the parameters used to measure this reactivity were inadequate to detect mild degrees of hyperkinetic response characterized by elevated catecholamines but no blood pressure or heart rate changes. These changes were not present in B's. It suggests that our measures of reactivity may be crude and insensitive enough to miss more subtle forms of arousal.

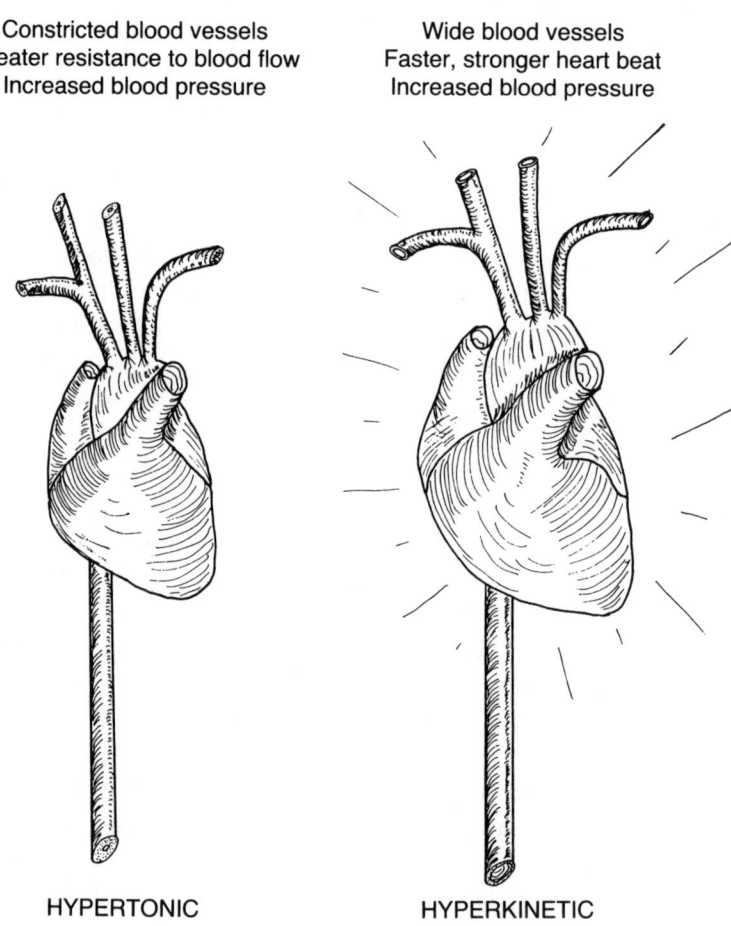

Figure 9

The hyperkinetic concept is interesting because it provides an opportunity to differentiate not only responses, but also their potential pathologic impacts. One could hypothesize a pattern of arousal in certain patients (i.e., A's) that involves less episodic vasoconstriction than labile or fixed hypertensives. The absence of this phenomenon conceivably could eliminate the chronic vascular alterations over time occurring in labile hypertensives, as well as kidney renin abnormalities. The arousal would have to seek another path to cause cardiovascular damage. The essential hypertensive has been easier to characterize as to the damage done to the vasculature over time; indeed the target organs of chronic hypertension are well documented to be kidney, brain, and heart. Labile hypertensives are assumed to invoke their risk via progression to fixed hypertension. There is, however, a suggestion that episodic reactivity, even the "mild" hyperkinetic type, is by virtue of catecholamine release potentially quite toxic in its own right, and provides an avenue via which Type A's might develop cardiovascular disease.

To place this into the perspective of daily life, it is important to recall that many daily events are or can be interpreted as harassing. The interplay between genetics and environment regarding stress responsiveness probably ultimately determines how we respond. We certainly cannot modify our genetics. It is not always possible to modify our environment, although there may be times when this would be appropriate. We can, however, alter our perceptions of environmental events, and, by so doing, perhaps alter our physiologic responses. This has important counseling and therapeutic implications.

We have begun to demonstrate why this is a desirable goal. We shall do so more definitively in the next chapter as we further elucidate the toxicity of catecholamine storm in both the context of the TABP and the labile hypertensive. We will strongly forge our link to coronary disease, and then begin consideration of what can be done to further our and our patients understanding of reactivity, and, most important, what, if anything, to do about it.

REFERENCES

1. Jorgensen, R., and Houston, B. K. Family history of hypertension, gender, and cardiovascular reactivity and stereotypy during stress. *J Behav Med*, 4:175–189, 1981.

2. Remington, R. D., et al. Circulatory reactions of normotensive and hypertensive subjects and of the childen of normotensive and hypertensive parents. *Am Heart J*, 59:58–70, 1969.
3. Rubenstein, E., and Federman, D. *Scientific American Medicine*. New York: Scientific American, 1984.
4. Hastrup, J. L., Light, K. C., and Obrist, P. A. Parental hypertension and cardiovascular response to stress in healthy young adults. *Psychophysiology*, 19:615–622, 1982.
5. Lawler, K. A., and Allen, M. T. Risk factors for hypertension in children: Their relationship to psychophysiological responses. *Psychosom Res* 23:199–204, 1981.
6. Steptoe, A., Melville, D., and Ross, A. Essential hypertension and psychological functioning: A study of factory workers. *Br; J Clin Psychol*, 21:303–311, 1982.
7. Falkner, B., et al. Effect of salt loading on the cardiovascular response to stress in adolescents. *Hypertension*, 3:195–199, 1981.
8. Steptoe, A., Melville, D., and Ross, A. Behavioral response demands, cardiovascular reactivity, and essential hypertension. *Psychosom Med*, 46:33–47, 1984.
9. Melville, D., and Raftery, E. B. Blood pressure changes during acute mental stress using the Oxford intra-arterial system. *J Psychosom Res*, 25:487–497, 1980.
10. Falkner, B., et al. Cardiovascular response to mental stress in normal adolescents with hypertensive parents. *Hypertension*, 1:23–30, 1979
11. Hjemdahl, P., and Eliasson, K. Sympatho-adrenal and cardiovascular response to mental stress and orthostatic provocation in latent hypertension. *Cli Sci*, 57:189s–191s, 1979.
12. Nestel, P. J. Blood pressure and catecholamine excretion after mental stress in labile hypertension. *Lancet*, 1:692–695, 1969.
13. Johnston, D. W., and Shaper, A. G. Type A behaviour in British men: Reliability and intercorrelation of two measures. *J Chron Dis*, 29:381–394, 1983.
14. Goldstein, D. Plasma norepinephrine during stress in essential hypertension. *Hypertension*, 3:551–556, 1981.
15. Lawler, J. E., et al. The effects of conflict on tonic levels of blood pressure in the genetically borderline hypertensive rat. *Psychophysiology*, 17:363–370, 1980.
16. Lawler, J. E., et al. Effects of stress on blood pressure and cardiac pathology in rats with borderline hypertension. *Hypertension*, 3:496–505, 1981.
17. Freidman, R., and Dahl, L. The effect of chronic conflict on the blood pressure of rats with a genetic susceptibility to experimental hypertension. *Psychosom Med*, 37:402–416, 1975.
18. Lorimer, A. R., et al. Blood pressure and catecholamine responses to "stress" in normotensive and hypertensive subjects. *Cardiovas Res*, 5:169–173, 1971.
19. Shapiro, A. P., Moutsos, S. E., and Krifcher, E. Patterns of response to noxious stimuli in normal, hypertensive, and diabetic subjects. *Jo Clin Inves*, 42:1890–1898, 1963.
20. Svensson, J. C., and Theorell, T. Cardiovascular effects of anxiety induced by interviewing young hypertensive male subjects. *J Psychosom Res*, 26:359–370, 1982

21. Hollenberg, N. K., Williams, G. H., and Adams, D. F. Essential hypertension: Abnormal renal vascular and endocrine responses to a mild psychological stimulus. *Hypertension*, 3:11–17, 1981.
22. Sapira, J. D., et al. Differences in perception between hypertensive and normotensive populations. *Psychosom Med*, 33:239–250, 1971.
23. Brod, J., et al. Circulatory changes underlying blood pressure elevation during acute emotional stress (mental arithmetic) in normotensive and hypertensive subjects. *Clin Sci*, 18:269–279, 1959.
24. Groen, et. al. Effects of experimental emotional stress and physical exercise on the circulation of hypertensive patients and control subjects. *Jo Psychosom Res*, 26:141–154, 1982.
25. Fredrikson, M., et al. Haemodynamic and electrodermal correlates of psychogenic stimuli in normotensive and hypertensive subjects. *Biol Psychol*, 15:63–73, 1982
26. Keane, T. M., et al. Are hypertensives less assertive? A controlled evaluation. *J Consult Clin Psychol*, 50:499–508, 1982
27. Sullivan, P., et al. Anxiety, anger, and neurogenic tone at rest and in stress in patients with primary hypertension. *Hypertension*, 3:II-119–II-123, 1981.
28. Braunwald, E. *Heart Disease: A Textbook of Cardiovascular Medicine*, 2nd ed. Philadelphia: W. B. Saunders, 1984.
29. Eich, R. H., et al. Hemodynamics in labile hypertension. *Am Heart J*, 63:188–195, 1962
30. De Mendonca, M., et al. Plasma catecholamines in conscious rats: Influence of sodium, stress and heredity. *Experentia*, 37:1087–1089, 1981
31. Several papers referenced in 32 (refs.) 3–5, p. 431).
32. Light, K. C., et al. Psychological stress induces sodium and fluid retention in men at high risk for hypertension. *Science*, 220:429–431, 1983.
33. Esler, M., et al. Mild high-renin essential hypertension: Neurogenic human hypertension? *N Engl J Med*, 296:405–411, 1977.
34. Folkow, B., and Rubenstein, E. H. The functional role of some autonomic and behavioral patterns evoked from the lateral hypothalamus of the cat. *Acta Physiol Scand*, 66:182–188, 1966.
35. Folkow, B., and Rubenstein, E. H. Cardiovascular effects of acute and chronic stimulations of the hypothalamic defence area in the rat. *Acta Physiol Scand*, 68:48–57, 1966.
36. Weiner, H., Singer, M., and Reiser, M. F. Cardiovascular responses and their psychological correlates. 1. A study in healthy young adults and patients with peptic ulcer and hypertension. *Psychosom Med*, 24:477–498, 1962.
37. Kalis, B., et al. Response to psychologic stress in patients with essential hypertension. *Am Heart J*, 53:572–577, 1957.
38. Hokanson, J. E., and Burgess, M. The effect of status, type of frustration, and aggression on vascular processes. *J Abnorm Soc Psychol*, 65:232–237, 1962.
39. Gambaro, S., and Rabin, A. I. Diastolic blood pressure responses following direct and displaced aggression after anger in high- and low-guilt subjects. *J Pers Soc Psychol*, 12:87–94, 1969.
40. Harburg, E., Erfurt, J. C., et al. Socio-ecological stress, suppressed hostility, skin color, and black-white male blood pressure: Detroit. *Psychosom Med*, 35:276–296, 1973.
41. Gentry, W. D., Harburg, E., and Hauenstein, L. Effects of anger expression/inhibition and guilt on elevated diastolic blood pressure in high/low

stress and black/white females. *Proc Am Psychol Assoc*, 115–116, 1973.
42. Harburg, E., Blakelock, E. H., and Roeper, P. J. Resentful and reflective coping with arbitrary authority and blood pressure: Detroit. *Psychosom Med*, 41:189–202, 1979.
43. Harburg, E., et al. Socio-ecological stressor areas and black/white blood pressure: Detroit. *J Chron Dis*, 26:595–611, 1973.
44. Gentry, W. D., Chesney, A. P., et al. Habitual anger-coping styles: 1. Effect on mean blood pressure and risk for essential hypertension. *Psychosom Med*, 44:195–201, 1982.
45. Alexander, F. Emotional factors in essential hypertension: Presentation of a tentative hypothesis. *Psychosom Med*, 1:173–179, 1939.
46. Cochrane, R. High blood pressure as a psychosomatic disorder: A critical review of the evidence. *Br J Soc Clin Psychol*, 10:61–72, 1971.
47. Elmadjian, F., Hope, J. M., and Lamson, E. T. Excretion of epinephrine and norepinephrine in various emotional states. *J Clin Endocrinol*, 17:608–620, 1957.
48. Von Euler, U. S. Quantitation of stress by catecholamine analysis. *Clin Pharmacol Ther*, 5:398–404, 1964.
49. Steptoe, A., and Ross, A. Psychophysiological reactivity and the prediction of cardiovascular disorders. *J Psychosom Res*2, 25:23–31, 1981.
50. Eliot, R. S., and Buell, J. C. The role of the CNS in cardiovascular disorders. *Hosp Prac*, 189–199, May 1983.
51. Williams, R. B., Lane, J. D., et al. Type A behavior and elevated physiological and neuroendocrine responses to cognitive tasks. *Science*, 218:483–485, 1982.

6

THE STORM BREAKS: CORONARY HEART DISEASE AND OTHER SEQUELAE

*T*he final common pathway linking stress to pathologic effects on the heart and vasculature in both the hypertensive and the Type A individual appears to be sympathomedullary arousal in response to environmental stimuli. If this is true, and the evidence of the last two chapters leads us in this direction, then the mind–body connection is made. Serum catecholamines are not seen to be universally elevated in these studies, but the manifestations of sympathetic activation have almost always been present. The reason for the discrepancy probably lies in the fact that catecholamines are released from sympathetic nerve terminals in minute amounts and are rapidly inactivated at the site of their release. Catecholamines, primarily epinephrine, secreted by the adrenal gland, are in essence hormones and circulate in far higher concentrations in the bloodstream (see Chapter 2). It is likely that the adrenal does not participate to the same degree in all instances of arousal, and sympathetic *nervous* activity (as opposed to hormonal) may be primarily responsible for the observed reactivity, a phenomenon very difficult to measure directly in intact organisms. Instead we infer its occurrence from the increases in blood pressure, pulse rate, etc., which are responses known to be mediated by this system.

We thus have demonstrated increased catecholamines or their physiologic correlates in A's and labile hypertensives, though in response to different stressors. We know that labile hypertensives over time appear to develop fixed high blood pressure, and we infer damage to coronary arteries based on a "wear-and-tear" hypothesis. We know there is not an increased incidence of fixed hypertension in Type A's, and therefore it is unlikely that intermittent arousal in response to stressors effects damage to the arteries in the same way that it does in the hypertensive population. We have suggested that the manifestations of sympathetic activation in A's may be different than in the hypertensive. Often subtle and hard to measure, it is the so-called hyperkinetic response. We introduced a third population of individuals, behaviorally distinct from A's, who also become physiologically aroused in response to nonphysical environmental stimuli. This is the so-called silent reactor, who may or may not be different from the labile hypertensive.

What we have yet to do is to tie the knot tightly between various patterns of reactivity in response to psychogenic stressors and damage to the heart and vasculature. The wear-and-tear hypothesis will not do for A's, at least not as neatly as it seems to for the hypertensive. We will therefore spend the remainder of this chapter discussing other consequences of the intermittent catecholamine storm.

We now examine in detail the toxicity of sympathomedullary arousal, mediated by adrenal hormonal stimulation or via sympathetic nervous activity. It is this toxicity that hyperreactors confront when the stressors in their lives arouse their physiology. Lest one gain the impression that once coronary heart disease is an established fact, the catecholamines can do no further harm, we will look at the consequences of sympathetic storm on the patient with clinical heart disease as well. Here we will find more clarity and agreement, and some interesting insights into the mechanisms of fear, anger, and sudden death.

We do not know for certain the initiating event of atherosclerotic lesions. We know that somehow blood clotting is involved, both because of the presence of clot in plaques, and because, rarely, blood clots can occlude arteries actuely, thus causing a heart attack without the presence of underlying plaques. We also suspect a role for calcium, scar tissue, and cholesterol, for much the same reasons. Spasm of arteries is clearly involved in certain cases of angina, and infarction as well. If we wish to understand the impact of sympathomedullary arousal on coronary heart disease, it is worthwhile to

Platelets are small packets of circulating clotting factors surrounded by a membrane. They are not true cells, but are fragments thereof, released from giant precursors in the bone marrow. When activated, they adhere to a surface, usually a damaged or irregular one, and initiate a cascade of biochemical reactions designed to form clots over the area. We alluded previously to the effect of epinephrine on platelets. There is little argument that these blood-clotting agents are activated by this hormone, which makes good teleologic sense of one is lacerated during fight-or-flight. However, the increased platelet stickiness might contribute to the formation of blood clots in the coronary arteries at the site of minor vascular injury. To test this hypothesis, animal studies have been done in which platelets were activated by the infusion of epinephrine or its analogs and in pigs were later found aggregated in the coronary arteries. Areas of cardiac muscle damage distal to the plugs were noted when the animal's hearts were examined at necropsy, suggesting that the platelets had occluded the vessels with resultant tissue death beyond the plugs from lack of oxygen.[1] To carry this a step further, drugs that are capable of inhibiting platelet aggregation were given to experimental animals prior to the infusion, and far less cardiac damage was seen in those animals as opposed to those that received the epinephrine infusions alone.[2] To ascertain whether these findings were related to an exogenous (given from without) drug effect of the infusion or were due solely to the catecholamines regardless of their source, rats were exposed to profound physical stress such as electric shock and hot water immersion, which stimulated their own catecholamines and platelet plugs similar to those seen in the other studies were found in small coronary arteries.[3,4] Certainly such evidence is preliminary, but it does strengthen the general hypothesis of the sympathomedullary contribution to coronary disease. The presumption of platelet involvement in atherosclerosis is strong enough among clinicians to warrant the virtually routine use of platelet-inhibiting drugs in patients who have had myocardial infarctions or warning strokes as a measure to prevent further thrombosis (clotting); indeed, certain groups of patients treated with these drugs (one of which is aspirin) have a decreased incidence of further infarctions than do controls.[5]

We can be a bit more definitive regarding the interaction of other coronary risk factors with stressful circumstances and presumed attendant physiologic arousal, most notably cholesterol. We are not sure just how elevated cholesterol contributes to CHD, but demographically it does, and it is present in atherosclerotic plaques. A recent study, much discussed in the lay press,[6] demonstrated that a reduction in serum cholesterol is accompanied by a reduction in the risk of heart disease. Several experimental studies[7-9] have shown an elevation of the serum cholesterol in response to epinephrine injections in animals. The most recent of these[7] took great care to use physiologic, as opposed to pharmacologic, doses and demonstrated a "significant" elevation (percentages not specified), presumably suggesting that the aroused state, accompanied by elevated catecholamines, induces an elevation in serum cholesterol.

Further, a host of studies, predominantly in humans, has demonstrated an elevation of the cholesterol in response to stressful circumstances. These are reviewed by Dimsdale[14] and show a range of 8–65 percent increases in cholesterol in response to various stressors, both naturally occurring and in the laboratory setting. The most profound increases were seen in medical students under examination stress, in novice fliers on aerobatic maneuvers, in certain types of military training, during stress interviews, and in various laboratory situations, such as anticipation of cold water immersion. Not all studies demonstrated significant increases, but of the 43 papers reviewed, 28 showed an increase, 11 no change, and four a decrease. Several generic problems inherent in these studies were discussed, including the datedness of much of the research, and hence of the biochemical assays used; the uncertainty of the time course of elevation of the cholesterol after stress; the different intervals, from minutes to days, used to assess the impact of the stressor on the serum measurement; and the duration and intensity of the stressor necessary to evoke the elevations. Nonetheless it is the conclusion of the reviewer that "most studies found that cholesterol increased from 8-65 percent above baseline under stressful conditions."

The significance of this may be somewhat different than the observation that elevated baseline cholesterol is a known classical risk factor for the development of coronary heart disease, and implies that cholesterol elevations, like blood pressure, may be a labile phenomenon in some individuals. We do not know whether episodic cholesterol elevations carry the same risk for coronary heart disease as do sustained elevations, nor do we have data on this process in A versus B individuals. However, one large study has demonstrated a higher cholesterol in Type A individuals, despite the fact that the risk factors are independent.[15]

In both of these instances, cholesterol and platelets, we again can only infer causal relationships among stressors, physiologic arousal, and biochemical and pathologic consequences. Fortunately for our inquiry, it is possible to measure more directly the impact of sympathomedullary activation on the heart and vasculature, both in experimental animals and in humans.

The catecholamines have repeatedly been shown to induce direct heart muscle (technically termed myocardial) damage in both humans and animals. It is clearly easier to study this directly in animals. In human beings we again must rely primarily on indirect evidence of cardiac damage to assess catecholamine toxicity. This is done via the electrocardiogram, a recording of the electrical activity in the heart muscle (Figure 10). In addition to demonstrating cardiac rate and rhythm, one is able to diagnose injury or death of heart muscle based on changes in the patterns of electrical activation of the tissue. One can even diagnose inadequate blood supply limited by an atherosclerotic plaque when the demand is increased by stress or exercise. This variant of the electrocardiogram, called a stress exercise or treadmill test, is one of the most useful noninvasive diagnostic tools available to clinicians and researchers. Much of the work we now explore draws its data and conclusions from electrocardiographic and stress test findings.

Let it be said at the outset that there is not universal agreement on the meaning and interpretation of many of the more subtle electrocardiogram changes used in research. The change we will deal with as an indicator of deleterious effects on a presumably normal heart in response to stress, termed ST-segment depression, has been held by some[10] to indicate an imbalance between blood supply and demand to heart muscle, a change that is not controversial when it occurs in the presence of coronary heart disease. The change consists of a dip in the electrical potential of the repolarizing heart muscle (see Figure 11). This would indicate, if not actually coronary narrowing, at least an imbalance, however, temporary, between supply and demand. However, subtle depression also has been termed a "nonspecific" change of uncertain significance. Most researchers interpret this change, along with variations in the height of the electrical waves (amplitude, see Figure 10), as indicators of catecholamine effect on the heart.[10–13]

We are for the moment interested in arousal-induced damage that might contribute to the development of coronary heart disease in a normal heart, and so will defer our discussion of electrocardiographic effects of stress on a heart with established coronary heart disease. For now, suffice it to say that despite the controversy, the abnormalities seen in the studies we are about to discuss are closely analogous to the abnormalities seen under catecholamine stress in patients afflicted with atherosclerosis of the coronary arteries, and the changes in those patients are unquestionably path-

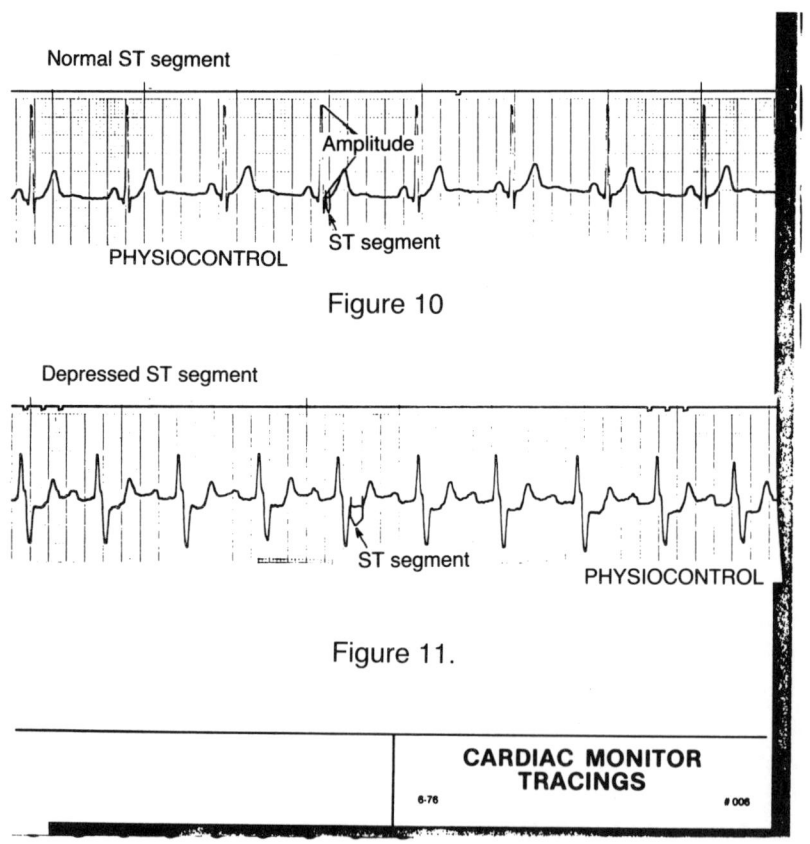

Figure 10

Figure 11.

ologic. It has also been shown repeatedly that exogenous epinephrine injections in normals cause ST depression.[13,16,17]

A study discussed previously in the context of A/B reactivity[10] pitted subjects against a computer in a competitive interactive strategy game and monitored the subjects' electrocardiograms. The Type A college students, with presumably normal hearts, displayed greater ST depression and diminished amplitude in response to the stressor than did their B counterparts suggesting catecholamine stimulation. Interestingly, there were no differences in heart rate (blood pressure was not measured). Here is another subtle manifestation of arousal not identified by classical measures that indicates a direct effect of the arousal on the target organ in which we are interested, and on the blood supply of that organ, the coronary arteries. Four older studies[13,18-20] describe similar electrocardiogram changes in response to psychic stress or trauma, some based on recall of past emotional events,[18] others on anecdotal case histories,[13,19] and one in response to hypnotically induced fear–pain–anxiety states,[20] again in individuals with presumably normal hearts.

Although we are not yet able to infer actual tissue damage to the arteries of heart muscle on the basis of these data, we do get closer, and are able to add another correlate of reactivity, a bit more sophisticated and specific, to our armamentarium. To look at exactly what catecholamines do to the heart, we must rely on autopsy studies, much as the platelet studies described above. Of course, our subjects are predominantly (but not exclusively) animals.

It has been known for almost 100 years that injections of epinephrine into experimental animals—such as rats, pigs, turtles, rabbits, hamsters, and dogs—are capable of directly damaging the heart.[21-24] The lesions produced are remarkably consistent across species, and consist of small areas of tissue death (necrosis), scarring, and bleeding into the muscle. Inflammation is common, and the changes vary directly in their intensity with dosage and frequency of administration. Because epinephrine and its analogs are used clinically to treat shock in critically ill patients, autopsies have been done in humans who received epinephrine infusions. Not surprising are lesions virtually identical to those found in experimental animals.[25-27] In addition there exists a rare disease in humans called pheochromocytoma, which is a tumor of the adrenal gland that produces large amounts of epinephrine. Patients dying of this disease have cardiac pathology similar to that of the animals described.[28,29]

A crucial link is provided by the comment of the author of a review of catecholamine toxicity[30] that "the striking similarity between the microscopic lesions induced by catecholamines and those seen after myocardial infarction has been recognized by many investigators."

As was the case with platelet aggregation, we find that catecholamines secreted by the organism are also capable of creating these cardiac lesions when large amounts are released during stressful circumstances. Raab studied wild and domestic rats faced with isolation, loud noises, and frustrating circumstances, and found the usual myocardial lesions much more frequently than in control animals.[31] A study was done in which pigs were paralyzed by a drug that left their conscious perception intact, so that they were unable to escape a threatening circumstance but were perfectly aware that a threat existed. The pigs were found to sustain profound cardiac damage, presumably in response to massive catecholamine discharge in the face of an inability to respond physically. In addition, 13 percent of the animals died suddenly, as discussed further later in the chapter.[32] Electrocardiographic changes accompanied the injury in most of these animals.

Finally, borderline hypertensive rats who were made quite hypertensive by an unresolvable conflict situation as discussed in the last chapter had the same myocardial lesions we have come to expect with catecholamines.[33]

None of this tells us how catecholamines might create CHD, but only that they damage the heart directly. Much discussion has ensued about *how* they do so, and it has been proposed, because of the similarities of pathology between catecholamine damage and a heart attack, that catecholamines kill heart muscle by disrupting blood supply, and hence starve the muscle for oxygen. This is felt to occur both because of platelet plugs and because of changes in blood flow induced by constriction of arteries.[27,34–36] So it would seem that an end result of coronary heart disease, myocardial infarction, can occur, at least in one form, by a parallel and not necessarily coexistent mechanism—catecholamine storm. The essential connection, however, eludes us still. Though we have considerable indirect evidence, we do not know if sympathomedullary arousal over time contributes directly to atherosclerosis.

What, then, are the effects of catecholamines on blood vessel walls? Large doses of epinephrine promote damage to blood vessels; necrosis, or death of portions of wall, calcium deposits, and hemorrhages into "plaques" in the aorta, the largest artery of the body, are seen in experimental animals. Unfortunately these lesions are rarely found in coronary arteries and do not contain cholesterol, which makes them not very analogous to coronary heart disease in humans. However, small, repeated doses of epinephrine do create a picture more characteristic of human atherosclerosis, both in location and nature.[30] In addition, patients dying of pheochromocytoma, the catecholamine-secreting tumor, also show lesions quite characteristic of early atherosclerosis.[30,37]

Are stressful circumstances, as opposed to exogenously administered catecholamines, sufficient to induce atherosclerosis in experimental animals? There is a small body of literature that addresses this issue. One example is a study of cholesterol-fed cockerels that demonstrated that the atherosclerotic process could be enhanced by placing the birds in an "unnatural" environment.[38]

Unfortunately for monkeys, they appear to be the animal model that mostly closely approximates the human condition. There are two studies, separated by 18 years, that deserve mention, as they tighten the bond between physiologic arousal and coronary heart disease. The first[38] was an attempt to induce atherosclerosis in one-year-old squirrel monkeys by feeding them elevated cholesterol diets and exposing them to an electric shock in a Skinner box that could be avoided by pressing a lever at a certain time. There were two control groups; one was placed in the box but not shocked, and the other was simply caged. Both groups restrained in the Skinner box for an hour a day developed significant coronary heart disease; the unmolested controls had none.

The second study, reported quite recently,[39] found that Cynomolgus monkeys could be divided into two groups, based upon their heart rate response to stressful stimuli. These differences were consistent among individuals over time and circumstance; that is, a high hot reactor reacted not only to the experimental stress, but also to the presence of the researcher in the room, unlike the low reactor who was apparently less stressed by the examiner's presence. The mean difference between the groups under stress was 37 beats per minute, although their baselines were the same it seems as if there are hot reactors among monkeys, too. All monkeys were fed a "moderately atherogenic" diet; that is, one designed, by virtue of elevated cholesterol content, to enhance the atherosclerotic process. Hot reactors had significantly greater atherosclerotic lesions in the coronary arteries at autopsy than did the low hot reactor responders. In addition, the high hot reactors exhibited "higher levels of contact aggression" than their counterparts. It would be redundant to emphasize the similarity to the Type A behavior pattern (TABP) and the hostility data of Chapter 4. This article is, in my view, one of the most definitive bits of evidence that intermittent sympathomedullary arousal in cardiovascular hyperreactors contributes directly to the atherosclerotic process.

We approach a potentially important clinical truth: Repeated episodes of sympathomedullary arousal seem capable of damaging the vasculature of the heart in a fashion quite similar to (or identical with) atherosclerosis. Let me reconstruct the scenario. A Type A or labile hypertensive undergoes episodic cardiovascular arousal in response to a variety of psychogenic stressors. Because no physical activity is called for, the vascular resistance stays high, with no increase of flow to working muscles. Instead the increased cardiac output batters the vessels, particularly at points of branching (where most CHD lesions occur). Minor breaches in the integrity of the vessel wall are overlaid by activated platelets that induce clot formation, and directly damage the wall further by means of certain enzymes released during the clotting process.[40] Cholesterol and other fats, whose concentrations in the blood are increased by epinephrine, are deposited in the damaged region, with scarring and calcium deposition taking place more gradually. Excessive proliferation of the muscle cells in the vessel wall, felt by some to contribute to the process, may be an attempt to protect downstream vessels, which are smaller but more fragile, from the intermittent or sustained hypertension. Direct damage to the muscle itself is a further consequence of the periodic catecholamine storms.

We thus synthesize, or attempt to synthesize, a working hypothesis based on the observed data. The challenge of future research in this area will be to develop ways of testing this premise, and being more definitive about the mechanisms involved. However, to a clinician, there comes a time when data must be acted upon because the evidence that the paradigm is essentially correct becomes overwhelming. The practitioner, who is quite different from the basic scientist, is eager to turn hard data to the advantage of his or her patient. As a practitioner I am led to the inescapable conclusion that there is truth and practical insight in all this, and that its implications for health are so profound that it must be acted upon.

For my colleagues or readers who remain somewhat skeptical, it is worth exploring briefly the impact of the catecholamines on a heart already afflicted with coronary disease, a topic of unquestioned clinical authenticity. These effects are dramatic and often fatal, as we shall see, and this should serve to emphasize the critical nature of sympathomedullary arousal and its contribution to disease processes. It will also dramatize the necessity for intervention.

We have noted previously that patients with coronary disease tend to be hyperreactors to various stressors. We assume that this hyperreactivity is mediated via sympathomedullary pathways, and hence via catecholamines. Certainly one would expect at least as much toxicity from these agents in a diseased heart as in a well one, and, as we shall see, probably significantly more. A common clinical test for the presence or severity of coronary heart disease is the exercise tolerance or stress treadmill test. The heart is stressed by exercise and the electrocardiogram is recorded, with ST depression at greater or less levels of cardiac work indicative of the severity of arterial obstruction. On the basis of the known reactivity of patients with established coronary heart disease to mental stress, a mental stress test has been proposed by several investigators. This test, using forced mental arithmetic or quiz interviews and recording the electrocardiogram, demonstrates ST depression in patients with coronary heart disease, generally correlating quite well with their exercise tolerance results.[41-43] ST depression was greater in patients with coronary disease than in controls in all of the studies, and executives with coronary heart disease demonstrated greater reactivity,[43] perhaps reminiscent of the Type A data (presuming many executives are Type A).

A recent study, reported in the British medical journal *The Lancet*, that utilized sophisticated imaging techniques showed that mental arithmetic was capable of inducing "silent" ischemia or oxygen lack without any symptoms of angina in 62 percent of 16 patients with known coronary heart disease. Thirty-seven percent had no accompanying ST depression.[44] This silent oxygen starvation was made manifest by subtle abnormalities detected by a nuclear imaging tool called positron tomography, and suggests that the routine tools for detecting ischemia are not sensitive enough for either physical or mental stress testing.

A real-life analog of these laboratory situations was demonstrated by recording electrocardiograms while the subject was driving an automobile on busy city streets.[45] Patients with known coronary heart disease had significantly greater ST depression during this task, so that the authors concluded: "Persons in whom angina is easily provoked while driving . . . should be advised not to drive."

Not all patients with coronary heart disease have positive mental stress tests. One group of researchers demonstrated that even in patients with the same extent of coronary heart disease by angiography, there were those who did not have positive mental stress tests despite positive treadmills.[41] This, again, suggests that there are subpopulations of patients with coronary disease who are more easily physiologically aroused by psychogenic stressors. This is intuitively sensible, and also points out again that one does not have to be a hyperreactor to have coronary disease. One would suspect that these individuals might be A's, former labile hypertensives, or the ill-defined silent hot reactor discussed previously. Regardless of their origins, however, these patients would be expected to be at increased risk from catecholamine toxicity superimposed on their coronary disease, because of the presumably frequent hormone storms they experience in response to psychogenic stress. One particularly nasty and frequently fatal consequence of intense sympathomedullary arousal in a diseased heart is arrythmia, or disorder of cardiac rhythm.

It is a well-known clinical principle of anesthesiologists and cardiologists that catecholamines sensitize a heart that is receiving inadequate oxygen to dangerous disorders of rythm. These disorders may precede or degenerate directly into cardiac arrest and subsequent sudden death. By its nature coronary heart disease results in limitation of oxygen delivery to the heart muscle under situations of increased demand. The severity of blockage determines the level of cardiac work necessary to create oxygen shortage, known as ischemia. The clinical symptom of angina, described in Chapter 3, is a frequent result. However, if ischemia is superimposed on a catecholamine storm (which by its increase in rate and force of cadiac contraction and hence cardiac work might have originally provoked the ischemia), the heart may become electrically unstable, the usual orderly progression of electrical impulses that result in synchronized beating may be disrupted, and cardiac arrest may occur (Figure 12).

Most of us have experienced palpitations, or the heart "turning over" in the chest. This is a manifestation of abnormal electrical excitability known as a premature contraction (Figure 13). Extra beats of this nature are common and of little clinical significance when they occur in isolation or infrequently. They may be stimulated by caffeine or other drugs in normal hearts and are self-limited and benign. In the presence of CHD, however, palpitations may be harbingers of sudden death.

Sudden death is responsible for the demise of more than 400,000 people annually in the United States.[46] Civilians are being trained in CPR in an attempt to diminish this mortality, but this has proved of minor efficacy. There is nothing new here. The phrase "scared to death" is a familiar one. Grief, intense anger, and even great joy have been implicated as causes of such catastrophies. History is replete with dramatic documentations of this phenomenon, as illustrated by the following excerpt from Engel's article on "Sudden and Rapid Death During Psychological Stress"[46]:

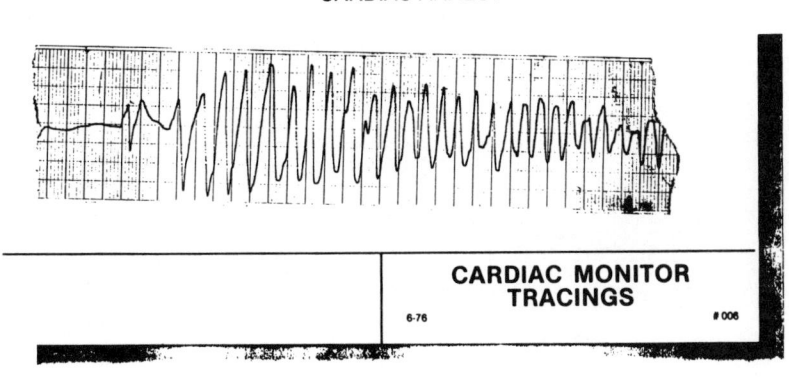

Figure 12.

THE STORM BREAKS

> Thus the Bible tells us that when Ananias was charged by Peter, "You have not lied to man but to God," he fell down dead; . . . Emporer Nerva is said to have died of a "violent excess of anger" against a senator who offended him, as did Valentinian while "reproaching with great passion" the deputies of a German tribe. Pope Innocent IV succumbed suddenly to the "morbid effects of grief on his system" soon after the disastrous overthrow of his army by Manfred, and King Philip V is said to have dropped dead when he realized the Spaniards had been defeated. Chilon of Lacedaemon is alleged to have died from joy while embracing his son who had borne away the prize at the Olympic games. [See article for references.]

Several modern-day studies have examined this issue in some detail, including retrospective analysis of the circumstances surrounding sudden death by examining newspaper accounts of the events. Engel in his study took this approach, and in some cases the news stories were enhanced by communication with relatives, attending physicians, or friends. These researchers were able to isolate 170 instances, primarily in the local press over a six-year period, that included details of the circumstances surrounding a sudden demise. All instances where suicide was even a remote consideration were excluded. Most deaths occurred within one hour of a presumably precipitating event. Eight situations were defined that accounted for all incidents: (1) impact of the collapse or death of someone close; (21 percent); (2) during a period of acute grief (within 16 days) (20 percent); (3) on threat of loss of someone close (9 percent); (4) during mourning or on an anniversary (3 percent); (5) on loss of status or self-esteem (6 percent); (6) in response to personal danger or threat of injury (27 percent); (7) after a danger

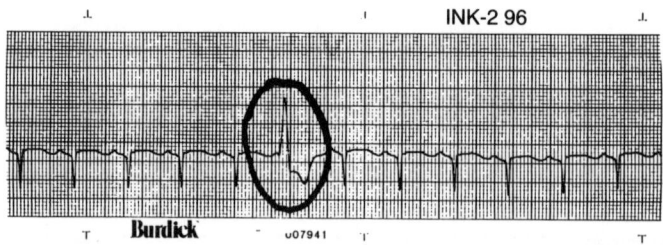

Figure 13.

was over (7 percent); and (8) upon reunion, triumph, or a happy ending (6 percent).

The age range of the individuals is interesting, with the mean age for men 45–55 and for women 70–75. Three children and four teenagers were included. A few examples are illustrative:

A 52-year-old man had been in close contact with his physician during his wife's terminal illness of lung cancer. . . . He died suddenly of a massive myocardial infarction the day after his wife's funeral.

A 40-year-old father slumped dead as he cushioned the head of his son lying injured on the street after a motorcycle accident.

A 52-year-old college president who prided himself on his support of black students died when a group of black students occupied the administration building.

A 55-year-old man died when he met his 88-year-old father after a 20-year separation; the father then dropped dead also.

A 75-year-old man, who hit the twin double for $1,683 on a $2 bet, died as he was about to cash in his ticket.

Similar reports abound, with numerous case histories cited in the medical literature[46,47]. Many deaths were in response to trivial incidents.

A 66-year-old man whose car broke down on the expressway died while trying to flag down passing motorists.

A 52-year-old city official died after giving a speech in a hotel; his predecessor had died under the same circumstances at the same hotel a year and a half earlier.

Most large studies demonstrate that approximately one-third of the victims of sudden death experienced stressful events on the day of their demise.[48]

A study of rescussitated survivors[48] found that anger was the predominant emotion preceding the event, and there did not appear to be any psychiatric abnormalities differentiating these people from those sustaining cardiac arrest who did not recall any particular predisposing circumstances.

Voodoo death, discussed by Walter Cannon,[49] who is best known for his description of the fight-or-flight response in the early 1940s, would appear to share similarities with the foregoing situations.

> A young negro on a journey lodged in a friend's house for the night. The friend had prepared for their breakfast a wild hen, a food strictly banned by a rule which must be inviolably observed by the immature. The young fellow demanded whether it was indeed a wild hen, and when the host answered "No," he ate of it heartily and proceeded on his way. A few years later, when the two met again, the old friend asked the younger man if he would eat a wild hen. He answered that he had been solemnly charged by a wizard not to eat that food. Thereupon the host began to laugh and asked him why he refused it now after having eaten it at his table before. On hearing this news the negro immediately began to tremble, so greatly was he possessed by fear, and in less than twenty-four hours was dead.

Again we must search for mechanisms. Surely not all of the individuals concerned had significant, or even any, coronary disease. One series indicated that approximately 65 percent of sudden deaths occur in individuals with coronary heart disease,[50] and another[51] found that death was related to coronary heart disease in 91 percent of males and 52 percent of females dying within an hour. Some patients died of other illnesses, such as strokes, and in many the cause of death was never ascertained. Some patients accurately predicted the time and circumstances of their own death, a phenomenon I have encountered more than once in clinical practice. Anecdotes, however, do not a model make. We must look a bit more rigorously at the problem.

The harbinger of sudden death, at least in the coronary care unit after a myocardial infarction, is the premature beat, or extrasystole (meaning extra contraction, see Figure 13). These extrasystoles may lead to ventricular fibrillation, the disorganized, chaotic electrical heart rhythm that results in sudden death, and is generally reversible only with electric shock delivered to the chest (Figure 12). In 1949 a study was reported wherein 12 patients with known extrasystoles were monitored while discussing topics "to which they were known to be sensitive." Extrasystoles increased in frequency as a result.[52]

This was, in essence, a mental stress test, and later studies using more sophisticated testing procedures have reported similar results. Lown et al.[53] found that 11 of 19 patients with preexisting heart disease and known electrical irritability (i.e., high frequency of premature beats) increased the frequency and severity of irritable cardiac manifestations by such psychogenic stressors. The automobile driving study demonstrated an increase of frequency of premature beats in five of 24 patients with coronary heart disease in addition to the ST changes while driving.

Statistically the combination of known coronary heart disease and preexisting extrasystoles significantly increases one's risk of ventricular fibrillation, and hence sudden death.[54,55] Premature beats in the absence of any other illness in one large study of 11,000 adults followed for 27 years were found to pose a small but significant increase in risk for sudden death.[56]

We must return to the catecholamines as a potential culprit in both premature beats and sudden cardiac death. We have mentioned the irritability induced by catecholamines in a heart receiving inadequate oxygen. We have discussed a variety of psychogenic stressors in whose setting sudden death seems to occur, particularly, although not exclusively, in the presence of CHD. We have also seen an increase in extrasystoles, particularly in diseased hearts, under stressful circumstances. For the anecdotes to have meaning, it would be useful to construct an animal model and test the impact of stress on cardiac irritability, and this has been done.

A number of studies have involved creating "artificial" coronary heart disease by tying off coronary arteries in dogs and pigs and subjecting these animals to various stressors. These studies have demonstrated that even minor stressors are capable of eliciting ventricular fibrillation[58-61] in these vulnerable hearts. Furthermore, it can be demonstrated that increasing sympathetic nervous activity to the heart lowers the electrical irritability threshold,[62] and administration of drugs that block the sympathetic nervous system renders animals resistant to fibrillation.[59,61] This, of course, has therapeutic implications, as discussed in the next chapter.

Numerous studies have attempted to delineate a psychological profile of coronary patients at risk for sudden death.[63-65] Dejection, depressive characteristics, and dissatisfaction with achievement were shown to have fairly strong predictive capabilities for sudden death in one prospective study. The last variable, also termed the "Sisyphus reaction" from the mythical character eternally pushing a rock up a hill and having it constantly roll back down, is considered an extreme of the TABP.

Patients in coronary care units seem to be at risk for ventricular fibrillation if they "react emotionally" to events around them in this often highly charged setting.[66]

As an intern, I specifically and vividly recall watching a very frightening movie late one night in the on-call room. I expressed to a colleague the fervent hope that one of my patients, a middle-aged woman who was recovering from a heart attack, was not watching it. At the climax of the movie, the cardiac arrest alarm was sounded—and it was indeed my patient, who had been watching the movie. Sadly, she did not survive the experience.

It certainly would seem that sympathomedullary arousal to psychogenic stressors may be fatal to patients with established CHD, and the mechanism would appear to be the interaction of the catecholamine storm with a diseased and irritable heart. However, this does not explain the fact that healthy children, adolescents, and experimental animals with normal hearts have also died from sudden and mysterious cardiac arrest, nor does it explain "voodoo death." It is possible, and likely, that massive catecholamine discharge can create cardiac arrest in a normal heart, as we have demonstrated that such discharges may be toxic in other ways. Another mechanism, however, elegantly formulated by Dr. George Engel, is worthy of consideration.

Dr. Engel believes that a counterpoint of the fight-or-flight sympathomedullary arousal exists, which he has termed "conservation withdrawal," and which has its analogs in the animal world as "sham death," hibernation, and estivation. This set of neurophysiologic changes, he proposes, serve to conserve energy, make the organism less conspicuous to predators, and promote withdrawal and disengagement from an environmental condition that cannot be fought or escaped. The response is mediated by the parasympathetic, or vegetative, nervous system, whose effects are essentially the opposite of sympathomedullary arousal. When an organism is subjected to intensely disorganizing, conflicting stimuli, the delicate reciprocity between the two systems fails, and evidence of activity of both sympathetic and parasympathetic nervous systems may be seen. In Engel's words:

> When the danger situation is one that has never been encountered; when environmental circumstances interfere with the normal response, as, for example, when an animal that normally meets danger by flight is physically restrained; or when a previous experience with the danger has established the futility of either response. The crucial psychologic variable is the degree of unresolvable uncertainty.

Fainting might be envisioned as falling into this category—for instance, when a man being inducted into the army is faced with a series of injections, and fleeing is inappropriate and hence inhibited. Fainting is not sudden death, but is always induced by a fall in blood pressure, and almost invariably is associated with a slow heart rate. The fall in blood pressure may be due to the fight-or-flight increase in blood flow to skeletal muscle, accompanied by a slow heart rate as a result of parasympathetic activation so that blood is "stolen" from the brain until the individual falls, and gravity reestablishes normal hemodynamics. Dr. Engels suggests that severe responses of this nature could, in fact, lead to cardiac arrest, even in a normal heart.[67] Several animal studies concur. The severe restraint that stress imposed on pigs, as we discussed earlier, was accompanied by sudden death, presumably secondary to a fatal arrythmias in 13 percent of these healthy animals. Other animals have died under similar stressful circumstances, particularly wild rats in captivity.[57]

Despite this it is important to emphasize again that the vast majority of instances of sudden death occur in patients with CHD, whether or not it has been clinically recognized. Other circumstances are rare.

From the discussions in the last three chapters, it should be clear that episodic sympathomedullary arousal to psychogenic stressors, whether in the Type A, the silent reactor, or the labile hypertensive, is potentially dangerous to the health of an organism, human or animal. The evidence—demographic, epidemiologic, experimental, and clinical—is quite convincing when considered in its entirety. However, as pointed out in Chapter 1, a world without stress is not possible, particularly in our modern corporate-academic Western society. We bear the burden of our genetic responses, certainly utilitarian in the face of physical threat, but largely obsolete in our lives of boardrooms and classrooms. We cannot, however, remove them as we would a useless appendix, but must learn to live with them. This is the topic of the next chapter.

REFERENCES

1. Jorgensen, L., Rowsell, H. C., Hovig, T., et al. Adenosine diphosphate-induced platelet aggregation and myocardial infarction in swine. *Lab Invest*, 17:616–644, 1967.
2. Haft, J. I., Gershengorn, K., Kranz, P. D., et al. Protection against epinephrine-induced myocardial necrosis by drugs that inhibit platelet aggregation. *Am J Cardiol*, 30:838–843, 1972.
3. Haft, J. I., and Fani, K. Intravascular platelet aggregation in the heart induced by stress. *Circulation*, 47:353–358, 1973.
4. Haft, J. I., and Fani, K. Stress and the induction of intravascular platelet aggregation in the heart. *Circulation*, 48:164–169, 1973.
5. Lewis, H. D., Jr., Davis, J. W., Archibald, D. G., et al. Protective effects of aspirin against acute myocardial infarction and death in men with unstable angina: Results of a Veterans Administration cooperative study. *New Engl J Med*, 298:289–293, 1983.
6. Lipid Research Clinics Program. The Lipid Research Clinics coronary primary prevention trial results I and II. Reduction in incidence of coronary disease and relationship of reduction in incidence of coronary disease to cholesterol lowering. *JAMA*, 251:351, 365, 1984.
7. Dimsdale, J. E., Herd, A. J., and Hartley, L. H. Epinephrine mediated increases in plasma cholesterol. *Psychosom Med*, 45:227–232, 1983.
8. –Drury, A. Immediate effects of epinephrine on phospholipides turnover and lipide partition in plasma, liver, and aorta. *Proc Soc Exp Biol Med*, 89:508–511, 1955.
9. Drury, A., and Moss, L. Experimental atherosclerosis: Effect of repeated injections of epinephrine on lipid partition of plasma and liver and aortic degenerative changes in intact rabbits. *J Gerentol*. 9:287–295, 1954.
10. Van Egeren, L. F., Fabrega, H., et al. Electrocardiographic effects of social stress on coronary-prone (Type A) individuals. *Psychosom Med*, 45:195–203, 1983
11. De Caprio, L., Cuomo, S., et al. R wave amplitude changes during stress testing. Comparison with ST segment depression and angiographic correlation. *Am Heart J*, 99:413–418, 1980.
12. Simons, H., and Hugenholtz, P. Gradual changes of the ECG wave during and after exercise in normal subjects. *Circulation*, 52:570–576, 1975.
13. Mitchell, B., and Shaprio, A. The relationship of adrenalin and T-wave changes to the anxiety state. *Am Heart J*, 48:323–330, 1954.
14. Dimsdale, J. E., and Herd, A. Variability of plasma lipids in response to emotional arousal. *Psychosom Med*, 44:413–430, 1982.
15. Rosenman, R., Brand, J., et al. Multivariate prediction of coronary heart disease during 8½ year followup in the Western Collaborative Group Study. *Am J Cardiol*, 37:902–910, 1976.
16. Hartwell, A., Burnett, J. et al. The effect of exercise and four commonly used

drugs on the normal human electrocardiogram. *J Clin Invest*, 21:409 412, 1942.
17. Clough, D. Effect of epinephrine on patients with "irritable heart." *Arch Intern Med*, 24:191–198, 1931.
18. Sigler, L. H. Emotion and atherosclerotic heart disease. I. Electrocardiographic changes observed on the recall of past emotional disturbances. *Br J Med Psychol*, 40:55–64, 1967.
19. Sigler, L. H. Abnormalities of the electrocardiogram induced by emotional strain: Possible mechanisms and implications. *Am J Cardiol*, 12:807–814, 1961.
20. Berman, R., Simonson, E., and Heron, W. Electrocardiographic effects associated with hypnotic suggestion in normal and coronary sclerotic individuals, 1967.
21. Raab, W. The pathogenic significance of adrenalin and related substances in the heart muscle. *Exp Med Surg*, 1:188–225, 1943.
22. Waters, I. L., and de Suto-Nagy, G. I. Lesions of the coronary arteries and great vessels of the dog following injection of adrenalin. *Science*, 111:634–635, 1950.
23. Nahas, G. G., Brunson, J. G., King, W. M., et al. Functional and morphologic changes in heart-lung preparations following administration of adrenal hormnones. *Am J Pathol*, 34:717–729, 1958.
24. Ferrans, V. J., Hibbs, R. G., et al. Histochemical and electron microscopical studies on the cardiac necrosis induced by sympathomimetic amines. *Ann NY Acad Sci*, 156:309–332, 1969.
25. Szakacs, J. E., and Cannon, A. L-norepinephrine myocarditis. *Am J Clin Pathoy*, 30:425–434, 1958.
26. Szakacs, J. E., and Mehlman, B. Pathologic changes induced by 1-norepinephrine. *Am J Cardiol*, 30:838–843, 1972.
27. Schenk, E. A., and Moss, A. J. Cardiovascular effects of sustained norepinephrine infusions. II. Morphology, *Circ Res*, 18:605–616, 1966.
28. Van Vliet, P. D., Burchell, H. B., and Titus, J. L. Focal myocarditis associated with pheochromocytoma. *N Engd J Med*, 272:1102–1108, 1966.
29. Kline, I. K. Myocardial alterations associated with pheochromocytomas. *Am J Pathoy*, 38:539–557, 1961.
30. Haft, J. I. Cardiovascular injury induced by catecholamines. *Prog Cardiovas Dis*, 17:73–86, 1974.
31. Raab, W., Chaplin, J. P., and Bajusz, E. Myocardial necroses produced in domesticated rats and in wild rats by sensory and emotional stresses. *Proc Soc Exp Biol Med*, 116:665–669, 1964.
32. Johansson, G., Jonsson, L., et al. Severe stress—Cardiopathy in pigs. *Am Heart J*, 87:451–457, 1974.
33. Lawler, J. E., Barker, G. F., et al. Effects of stress on blood pressure and cardiac pathology in rats with borderline hypertension. *Hypertension*, 3:496–505, 1981.
34. Maling, H. M., and Highman, B. Exaggerated ventricular arrythmias and myocardial fatty changes after large doses of norepinephrine and epinephrine in unanesthetized dogs. *Am J Physioly*, 194:590–596, 1958.
35. Ferrans, V. J., Hibbs, R. G., Black, W. C., et al. Isoproterenol-induced myocardial necrosis. A histochemical and electron microscopic study. *Am Heart J*, 68:71–90, 1964.

36. Handforth, C. P. Isoproterenol-induced myocardial infarction in animals. *Arch Pathol*, 73:161–165, 1962.
37. Hueper, W. C. Arteriosclerosis. *Arch Pasthol*, 38:245–285, 1944.
38. Lang, C. M. Effects of psychic stress on atherosclerosis in the squirrel monkey. *Proc Soc Exp Biol*, 126:30–34, 1967. (See reference 3, Pick et al.)
39. Manuck, S. B., Kaplan, J. R., and Clarkson, T. B. Behaviorally induced heart rate reactivity and atherosclerosis in Cynomolgus monkeys. *Psychosom Med*, 45:95–107, 1983.
40. Mills, D. C. B., Robb, J. A., and Roberts, G. K. The release of nucleotides, 5-hydroxytryptamine and enzymes from human blood platelets during aggregation. *J Physioly* (London), 195:715–729, 1968.
41. Specchia, G., de Servi, S., Falchone, C., et al. Mental stress testing in patients with coronary artery disease. *Am Heart J*, 108:57–63, 1984.
42. Sime, W. E., Buell, J. C., and Eliot, R. S. Cardiovascular responses to emotional stress (quiz interview) in post-myocardial infarction patients and matched control subjects. *J Hum Stress*, 6:39–46, 1980.
43. Schiffer, F., Hartley, L. H., et al. The quiz electrocardiogram: A new diagnostic and research technique for evaluating the relation between emotional stress and ischemic heart disease. *Am J Cardiol*, 37:41–47, 1976.
44. Taggart, P., Gibbons, D., and Somerville, W. Some effects of motor car driving on the normal and abnormal heart. *Br Med Jl*, 4:130–134, 1969.
45. Deanfield, J. E., et al. Silent myocardial ischemia due to mental stress. *Lancet*, 2:1001–1004, 1984.
46. Engel, G. L. Sudden and rapid death during psychological stress: Folklore or folk wisdom? *Ann Intern Med*, 74:771–782, 1971.
47. Harvey, W. P., and Levine, S. A. Paroxysmal ventricular tachycardia due to emotion: Possible mechanism of death from fright. *JAMA*, 150:479–480, 1952.
48. Reich, P. How much does stress contribute to cardiovascular disease? *J Cardiovas Med*, July 1983.
49. Cannon, W. B. "Voodoo" death. *Am Anthropol*, 44:169–181, 1942.
50. Kuller, L., Lilienfield, A., and Fisher, R. Epidemiological study of sudden and unexpected death in adults. *Medicine*, 46:341–361, 1967.
51. Spain, D. M., Bradis, V. A., and Mohr, C. Coronary atherosclerosis as a cause of unexpected and unexplained death. An autopsy study from 1949–1959. *JAMA*, 174:384–388, 1960.
52. Stevenson, I. P., Duncan, C. H., and Wolf, S. Life situations, emotions, and extrasystoles. *Psychosom Med*, 11:257–272, 1949.
53. Lown, B., and DeSilva, R. A. Roles of psychologic stress and autonomic nervous system changes in provocation of ventricular premature complexes. *Am J Cardiol*, 41:979–985, 1978.
54. Chiang, B. N., Perlman, L. V., et al. Relationship of premature systoles to coronary heart disease and sudden death in the Tecumseh epidemiologic study. *Ann Intern Med*, 70:1159–1166, 1969.
55. Pell, S., and D'Alonzo, C. A. Immediate mortality and five year survival of employed men with first myocardial infarction. *N Engl J Med*, 270:915–918, 1964.
56. Lyle, A. M. Coronary diseases as an underwriting problem. *Trans Soc Actuaries*, 15:324, 1963.
57. Hofer, M. A. Cardiac and respiratory function during sudden prolonged immobility in wild rodents. *Psychosom Med*, 32:633–647, 1970.

58. Lee, K. T., Lee, W. M., et al. Experimental model for study of "sudden death" from ventricular fibrillation or asystole. *Am J Cardioly*, 32:62–73, 1973.
59. Skinner, J. E., Lie, J. T., et al. Modification of ventricular fibrillation latency following coronary artery occlusion in the conscious pig. The effect of stress and beta-adrenergic blockade. *Circulation*, 51:656–667, 1975.
60. Lown, B., Verrier, R., and Corbalan, R. Psychologic stress and the threshold for repetitive ventricular response. *Science*, 182:834–836, 1973.
61. Matta, R. J., Lawler, J. E., and Lown, B. Ventricular electrical instability in the conscious dog: Effects of psychologic stress and beta adrenergic blockade. *Am J Cardiol*, 38:594–598, 1976.
62. Verrier, R. L., Thompson, P. L., and Lown, B. Ventricular vulnerability during sympathetic stimulation: Role of heart rate and blood pressure. *Cardiovas Res*, 8:602–610, 1974.
63. Bruhn, J. G., Paredes, A., et al. Psychological predictors of sudden death in myocardial infarction. *J Psychosom Res*, 18:187–191, 1974.
64. Bruhn, J. G., Chandler, B., and Wolf, S. A psychological study of survivors and non-survivors in myocardial infarction. *Psychosom Med*, 31:8–19, 1969.
65. Wolf, S. Central autonomic influences on cardiac rate and rhythm. *Mod Concepts Cardiovas Dis*, 38:29–34, 1969.
66. Wolf, S. Psychosocial forces in myocardial infarction and sudden death. In L. Livi (ed.), *Society, Stress and Disease*, Vol. I. New York: Oxford Press, 1971, pp. 324–330.
67. Engel, G. L. Psychologic stress, vasodepressor (vasovagal) syncope, and sudden death. *Ann Intern Med*, 89:403–412, 1978.

7

UNCORKING THE BOTTLE: DOES IT MATTER?

What can we do? Can we modify our physiology, our physical nature, to cope differently with the demands of our world and perhaps reduce the risk of vascular damage from the pent-up storm in a bottle? Should we release the storm, in fury, at our bosses, at our competitors, at those who challenge or confront us, and perhaps react physically in our genetically endowed fight-or-flight mode? This would uncork the bottle, give the thundering heart a motive for its frantic pumping—and probably land us in jail for violent antisocial behavior or disturbing the peace. Or can we in some way soothe the beast, placate the roiling waters in the blood vessels, perhaps perceive ourselves and our human condition differently so that the meaning of the challenges, their significance, and their ability to trigger our physiology are altered in some fundamental way? Is this possible, and if it is, will it reduce the risk of cardiovascular disease? It is these questions that will occupy us for the remainder of this book.

Preceding chapters have demonstrated, not without controversy, that there is a behavior pattern termed "A" associated with sympathomedullary arousal to environmental challenge, and that it possesses an increased risk for the development of coronary heart disease at least equal to that of smoking cigarettes, being hypertensive, or having an elevated cholesterol level. Within this population it appears that those who possess certain components of the pattern, such as hostility, are perhaps most at risk. There is another population of intermittent reactors, the labile hypertensives, which is at risk for the development of essential hypertension and its protean cardiovascular pathologies, including CHD. A third population of patients with established CHD who are not necessarily A, but who are hyperresponders to psychogenic stress, may be predisposed to sudden cardiac death, among other catecholamine toxicities. We have suggested, moreover, that there is probably a fourth population of "silent hot reactors" who are similar to the third group but without overt coronary disease. This group is clearly the most poorly defined and understood. The basis for the damage caused to the heart and vascular tree in all of these instances seems to lie in the excessive sympathetic nervous and hormonal discharge in the face of psychogenic stress. Interventions, then, could be aimed at (1) blocking sympathomedullary arousal by preventing nervous and hormonal discharge biochemically (sympathetic blockade), (2) reducing the excitability or sensitivity of the system (tranquilization), (3) giving the discharge appropriate physical outlets, (4) avoiding the stimuli that activate the system; or (5) altering perception or changing the perceived significance of stimuli so that they no longer are capable of eliciting sympathomedullary arousal.

However, first we must be convinced that it matters. Most of the therapeutic interventions we will review are time consuming, and many involve significant life-style changes. And as we know, the Type A has other things to do with his or her time. We must be convinced that change is possible, and that such change is accompanied by a significant reduction in risk of cardiovascular disease.

The risk factor most intensively studied and most hotly debated is the efficacy of blood pressure control in preventing the sequelae of sustained hypertension: heart attack, hypertensive heart disease, stroke, and kidney disease. Let us begin there. We will then proceed to consider alteration of the Type A behavior pattern (TABP) and its potential risk-modifying impact.

There is little debate or doubt that treatment of moderate to severe hypertension (diastolic blood pressure 105–129) is capable of at least retarding, and at best preventing, vascular disease, and of prolonging life and health. This determination arose from a study presented by the Veteran's Administration in the late 1960s and early 1970s, [1,2] which found a significant reduction in "morbid events," specifically stroke and heart failure, in middle-aged men upon treating their moderate to severe hypertension with medication. The numbers of "mild hypertensives" were small, and the results, though not statistically significant, followed a similar trend. There wasl, despite this, no reduction in the frequency of myocardial infarction by such therapy. However, many of the men entering the study were felt to have already sustained significant vascular damage, and had significant atherosclerosis. Nonetheless, differences between treated and untreated men were marked enough that it became the standard of care to detect and treat hypertension aggressively, and the study fostered many blood pressure educational and community screening programs. The changes have been many—witness the altered pattern of awareness of hypertension since the early 1960s, when a study showed 50 percent of hypertensives aware of their condition, 25 percent treated, and only 12 percent controlled,[3] compared to a 1980-1981 survey in Minneapolis-St. Paul[4] in which 76.1 percent of patients were aware and controlled, and only 6.6 percent previously undiagnosed at the time of the survey. Other surveys in New York and California are similarly impressive.[3]

The situation with the mild hypertensive is not nearly so clear. We mentioned that *mild* hypertensives (diastolic 90–105) were not heavily represented in the VA group, and hence the data did not reach statistical significance. In the general population, however, the situation is very different, with estimates of the number of patients with this entity ranging upward of 40 million.[5] It is around this group that the controversy turns. Let us see what all the fuss is about. There are three recent large-scale studies of thousands of men and women with mild hypertension, and it will be interesting and instructive to look briefly at the results of each, as well as their interpretation. Conclusions obviously could influence a large segment of the population. Bear with the details, for it is upon these that treatment recomendations for millions are based. Deciding whether or not to treat the mild hypertensive (or to be treated if you fall into this category) is a crucial decision that makes working through the research imperative.

The first was published in 1979. It compared the effects on total mortality of intensive systematic blood pressure control in special clinics with routine community-based medical care in 10,940 men and women over a five-year period.[7] Of these patients 71.5 percent were defined as "mild" according to the criteria. The study, termed the Hypertension Detection and Followup Program (HDFP), demonstrated consistently better blood pressure control in the intensive-care, or stepped-care, group, and an overall 17 percent reduction in mortality as compared with the community-treated patients. When mild hypertensives were considered separately, the differences were even more marked, with a 20 percent lower death rate in this group. Indeed, this was the *only* group in which the differences were considered statistically significant.

In breaking this mortality down by cause, it was determined that most of the patients succumbed to cardiovascular diseases, specifically stroke and heart attack. There were 45 percent lower deaths from strokes and 46 percent fewer deaths from myocardial infarction in the intensively treated mild hypertensives.

It is instructive to look at the absolute numbers involved here. Over the five-year study period, 768 patients died—349 in the stepped-care group and 419 in the community group. Therefore, there were 70 excess deaths in the latter group. Of these, 60 of the victims were mildly hypertensive. And of the 60 patients, 17 died of noncardiovascular, and presumably nonhypertension-related, disease. Causes of death varied from accidents and homicides to cancer, respiratory ailments, and infectious diseases. The absolute difference in mortality due to hypertension-related disease, therefore, was 43 mildly hypertensive patients from a total sample size of 7825, or 0.5 percent. Although this does not sound impressive, let us keep this number in mind, as we shall return to it as we explore the ways in which the medical community interprets data and pronounces treatment mandates.

The second study originated in Australia and appeared in 1980.[8] This work was a bit "purer" in the sense that all patients were mildly hypertensive, few had already established cardiovascular disease (not so in the HDFP), and the control group was untreated (except for receiving an inactive placebo). The group included 3427 men and women, who were followed over four years for both mortality and morbidity (the latter defined as illness presumed to result from hypertension, such as nonfatal strokes or heart attacks). Mild hypertensives were somewhat more liberally defined, with diastolic blood pressures of 95–110 needed to qualify. Only two-thirds of the initially enrolled patients continued either their active or placebo therapy until they had suffered a morbid event, died, or completed the four-year study period. The characteristics and numbers of dropouts were similar in the two groups, and so were felt not to bias the results.

As expected, treated patients enjoyed superior blood pressure control, with 64 percent of the active group maintaining diastolic blood pressures of less than 90, compared with 25 perent of the placebo patients. Of the placebo patients, 198 experienced progression fo their hypertension to a more severe range, whereupon they were treated, whereas only four of the treated group progressed. As in the HDFP study, there was a significant reduction in mortality, by two-thirds, due in large part to fewer cardiovascular deaths. There were half the number of nonfatal strokes in the treated group, with little difference in the incidence of nonfatal heart attacks. Differences in fatal heart attacks were just short of statistical significance. It is also worthy of note that the occurrence of all morbid or fatal end points correlated well with increasing blood pressure levels.

The authors point out that there were comparatively far fewer deaths in this group over the four years than in the HDFP study, presumably because the patients were healthier at entry.

Let us again look at the absolute numbers involved. Of the 2218 patients finishing the study, 28 patients died, 11 of noncardiovascular causes. Thirteen of the remainder were from the placebo group, four from the active. Therefore, there was 0.4 percent total excess mortality from hypertension-related disease. Nonfatal cardiovascular events numbered 190, of which 82 were in the active group and 108 in the placebo—a difference of 26, or 1 percent.

Both of these research groups showed that mild hypertensives should be treated, and treated vigorously. So how can something so apparently clear cut be so hotly debated? Conflict arose with the publication of the third study, in 1982, termed the Multiple Risk Factor Intervention Trial (MRFIT).[9]

The MRFIT attempted the somewhat heroic task of simultaneously attempting to modify three major cardiovascular risk factos—smoking, high cholesterol, and hypertension—in 12,866 high-risk males aged 35–57. The study was structured similarly to the HDFP, in the sense that patients were randomized between community-based care and special intervention clinics. The study period was seven years, during which patients were given counseling for cigarette smoking, dietary advice, and intensive hypertension treatment at the clinics.

The resulting data are a bit of a morass, but several findings are of direct interest to our inquiry. There were no statistically significant differences in overall mortality between the two groups. Overall, the hypertensive population demonstrated no benefit from the special intervention, with virtually identical total death rates exhibited. What was particularly distressing to these researchers, and the seat of the subsequent controversy, was an excessive mortality of 27 patients among hypertensive males in the intensive treatment group who entered the study with an abnormal electrocardiogram as compared with males in the community group with similar abnormalities. 15 of these deaths were cardiac related. To break this down still further, the majority of these deaths occurred in individuals with blood pressures in the 90–99 range. On the other hand, men with normal cardiograms in the special treatment group fared *better* than their counterparts, with 14 fewer deaths.

Why would more intensively treated hypertensives with abnormal electrocardiograms fare worse than men with the same abnormalities who were less intensively treated? This is the question that has changed the universal "Thou shalt treat the mildly hypertensive" mandate. The logical explanation would seem to revolve around some toxicity inherent in the intensive treatment. Certain antihypertensive medications, particularly the diuretics, or "fluid pills," can deplete the body of potassium, an essential salt. Several studies have demonstrated that such a depletion renders the heart more susceptible to premature beats,[10,11] particularly in the presence of elevated levels of epinephrine.[12] One could envision how a patient with an abnormal electrocardiogram, and hence perhaps already at risk for dangerous arrythmias, could have such a risk potentiated by diuretics, particularly when under stress. Unfortunately for this theory, both groups were given diuretics, although the data presented were not detailed enough to indicate whether the patients who died were more likely to have received them. Furthermore, the excess mortality was from all causes, not just coronary disease. It is also worth mentioning that diuretics are known to elevate serum cholesterol.

The patient with hypertension, as well as the treating physician, is left somewhat confused by all of this. Editorials in the medical literature have championed one or the other position, with no clear concensus on the horizon. But let us look closer at both the tangibles and the intangibles, as our labile hypertensives certainly will tend to become mild, and we must know what to do. Furthermore, one must take a stand regarding whether or not encourage mild hypertensives to pursue therapy.

One "no-treat" editorial published in the *Annals of Internal Medicine*, a journal widely read by internists,[13] points to the MRFIT data and says: "The patients with entry diastolic blood pressures between 90 and 94 who received antihypertensive therapy had higher mortality and morbidity than those who were treated less vigorously." This statement contains two errors. First, morbidity was not even addressed in this study, and second, the excess mortality was seen only among those men who had an abnormal electrocardiogram, as we have just discussed. The same writer further comments on the HDFP data: "If we consider the data in simple terms, for every 100 patients with mild hypertension, 1.3 had a definite benefit over a five-year period and 98.7 did not."

The fundamental problem here seems to be a combination of inadequate knowledge of the studies in question and a game of numbers in which some essential bits of information from these studies are overlooked. Both the HDFP and the MRFIT studies measure only mortality, and both do so over a relatively short time span. Consequences of hypertension may develop over the course of years, and so not be apparent from mortality statistics over a five- to seven-year follow-up. The comment that only 1.3 patients of every 100 had a definite benefit simply means that these people did not die during this period. It says nothing about other complications of the disease, and the efficacy of treatment in preventing them. Furthermore, if we look solely at mortality data and extrapolate these 1.3 per 100 saved lives to the 40 million mild hypertensives in the United States alone, we will save 520,000 lives in five years. I would be somewhat more conservative and recall that the excess mortality of HDFP was 0.5 percent; thus the number saved would be 200,000 over that period. Gifford,[3] in a counterpoint "pro-treat" editorial, arrives at 325,000, using a different method of calculation. Surely this is not inconsequential.

Gifford also points out that the greatest reduction in mortality in the HDFP study occurred in the mildest hypertensives (blood pressure 90–94) who had no evidence of "target organ" (heart, blood vessels, kidneys, eyes) damage from hypertension. Once target organ damage was present, mortality increased in both groups by a factor of four, although the special-care group still fared better. Surely the longer hypertension is present, the more likely it is that damage will occur in target organs. As Dr. Gifford asks: "What other evidence do we need to conclude that in patients with mild hypertension, treatment should be considered early, and certainly before damage to target end-organs has occurred?"

We have seen that untreated hypertension does progress to more severe stages, as witnessed by the Australian study.

As for the MRFIT data, Gifford points out a rather glaring inconsistency. He notes that, for unexplained reasons, hypertensive patients in the community care group who had abnormal electrocardiograms had a *lower* mortality than hypertensive patients in the same group with normal electrocardiograms. The numbers are of a lesser order of magnitude than the adverse mortality data; nonetheless the finding is unexplained, and counter to the findings that have stirred the pot so thoroughly. Why would patients with normal electrocardiograms have a higher death rate than those whose tracings suggested the presence of disease? This renders the studies' other conclusions suspect.

I treat the mild hypertensive, and summarize my reasons for doing so as follows:

1. The HDFP and Australian studies, designed to look specifically and only at hypertension, are reasonably unequivocal in their support of the "to-treat" position.

2. Mortality-only data may well overlook target organ damage and any slow progression of vascular disease in time frames exceeding those of all of the studies done to date.

3. Not only do the MRFIT data have inconsistencies and multiple variables, but they refer to patients known to be at high risk from a variety of factors. Even if the MRFIT data are accepted, patients with normal electrocardiograms appear to benefit from therapy, and these patients are likely to be healthier at baseline.

4. It is interesting to note that the MRFIT community treatment

and special intervention groups both experienced lower overall mortality than risk factor analysis based on demographic risk factor data would have suggested. A population corresponding in size and risk factor frequency to the community group of MRFIT would be expected to sustain 442 deaths in six years, including 187 from coronary heart disease. This group sustained only 219, with 104 from coronary heart disease.[9] This suggests that intervention even in the community-based group was successful in staving off mortality. One must remember that the thought among practicing physicians caring for the community group was probably based on the VA and HFDP studies, both of which supported rather aggressive treatment. Indeed, the differences in blood pressure between the two MRFIT groups at the end of the study was quite small (3.1 mmHg) and both groups showed excellent control of their blood pressure overall. I do not accept the MRFIT data as a mandate not to treat.

Most editorials note the fact that even without treatment a certain percentage of patients will demonstrate a spontaneous *decrease* in their blood pressures to normal levels after initial screening. They offer this as a reason to withhold therapy for several months to determine if the hypertension is sustained. This is not unreasonable, nor is the suggestion that nonpharmacologic measures such as salt restriction, exercise, or relaxation techniques be employed initially. My objection to comments that demean the significance of mild hypertension is that they lessen the commitment of the physician to treat these patients, regardless of the modality employed. In the next chapter, we discuss the efficacy of nonpharmacologic interventions, and whether they are worth the time and inconvenience inherent in many of them.

It is likely that many of the patients whose blood pressures diminish over time without therapy are labile hypertensives or hot reactors who adapt to the stress of blood pressure measurement in a clinical setting, and no longer undergo arousal when the measurement is being made. This, of course, tells us little about how they respond to the stresses of their daily lives, and whether hypertensive response to those stressors is an important risk factor for disease, and so should be treated.

A rather pivotal piece of research addresses this issue. We have mentioned the "target organ" concept several times, and the fact that one of these target organs is the heart. When the blood pressure is elevated, the heart must work harder to pump against the increased resistance in the blood vessels, a phenomenon called afterload.'' Consequently it hypertrophies, or thickens, much like the biceps of a weight lifter. This "ventricular hypertrophy," which can be detected by the electrocardiogram and ultrasound studies, ultimately can lead to pump failure, a sequence termed "hypertensive heart disease." A study reported in the cardiology journal *Circulation* demonstrates that the presence of cardiac hypertrophy was only weakly related to baseline blood pressures recorded at home or in a clinic, even if these were elevated, but related strongly and consistently to blood pressure measured at work. Blood pressures measured at home on a workday showed a substantial but somewhat weaker relationship, whereas in unemployed individuals and in patients who chose to have pressures measured on weekends the relationship was essentially absent.[14] Interestingly and not surprisingly, blood pressure readings in the same individuals were consistently higher at work and in the clinic than at home—cardiovascular hyperreactivity, we would term it.

This would seem to substantiate the hypothesis that even labile hypertension can cause damage, and daily stressors and the response to them can create real disease. At this point it would be premature to treat all labile or mild hypertensives with medications, at the least because such medications are not innocuous; in the next chapter some nonpharmocologic alternatives are explored. Suffice it to say now that hypertension—mild, and probably labile—*is* a significant threat to health, that it must be addressed, and that treatment does lower risk.

Hypertension can be treated physiologically; that is, medications can alter the vascular tone, cardiac force, or fluid volumes in the vessels, though this may not always be the optimal approach. Confronting a behavior pattern such as the TABP from a treatment perspective would seem to be a very different proposition. It has been suggested[15] that there are two general approaches to this problem: behavioral and cognitive. The first consists of interventions designed to alter or blunt sympathomedullary arousal, such as relaxation techniques, or even medications. The second is concerned with perceptual alterations, so that the awareness of stressors, their significance to the individual, and theoretically one's subsequent physiologic responsiveness, are altered. Because we do not really understand what triggers the hypertensive reaction, and the preliminary data of Chapter 6 suggest that the stimuli are more general and of a milder nature than might be assumed, a cognitive approach toward this entity is somewhat harder to pursue. Treatment for hypertension, then, is primarily in the first category: blunting physiology. Studies dealing with alteration of the TABP have followed both approaches. It is their success in modifying cardiovascular risk that we will now address.

In the late 1970s, several small studies reported diminution of the TABP according to Jenkins Activity Survey scores and self-report in patients without manifest coronary artery disease.[15-17] All were short-term (three- to 14-week) interventions utilizing both behavioral and cognitive approaches, with one study comparing the two.[16] Researchers in the latter case were able to demonstrate a decrease in cholesterol and blood pressure regardless of the modality employed, although this was not confirmed by others.[17] Sample sizes were small, and though six-month follow-ups were encouraging, results, by the study group's own admissions, were far from definitive.

What was most heartening was that patients were amenable to change, and that, at least in the short term, change was possible. One research group,[16] upon advertising for potential subjects, was overwhelmed by the response. Interestingly, almost all of the respondents were judged to be "A" by a screening interview, which tells us something about the accuracy of their self-appraisal.

The only study systematically to address CHD risk modification by changing Type A behavior was recently reported by Dr. Meyer Friedman, whom we have already mentioned as perhaps the most prominent researcher in the field.[18] This began with a group of 1035 post-myocardial-infarction men and women from the San Francisco area who were divided randomly into two groups. One group received group cardiologic counseling consisting of traditional dietary and exercise advice, drug compliance encouragement, and discussions of general fears and anxieties with no mention of the TABP (270 patients). The other group consisted of 60 small classes that received both the above treatment and intensive Type A behavioral counseling, including cognitive and behavioral components (592 patients). Twenty-two patients were excluded because previous myocardial infarction could not be clearly documented. The remaining 151 were nonrandomly placed in a third group, to be examined yearly by the researchers, but not included in any formal counseling beyond what they might receive from their own physicians. Members of this group were unable, for various reasons, to attend enough of the counseling sessions to participate in the randomization. Type A behavior was assessed by three separate questionnaires and the Structured Interview, and patients remained in counseling for three years. Incidents of recurrent fatal and nonfatal heart attacks were compared among the the groups. All baseline characteristics, (height, weight, presumed severity of coronary disease, presence of severity of other risk factors, and Type A scores) were remarkably similar in the three groups.

Motivation, it would seem degenerated incrementally over the three-year period, with 97 withdrawals from traditional group counseling and 200 from the Type A modification group. Almost all of these patients continued their yearly examinations, however.

Of the patients completing the Type A counseling, 31.7 percent exhibited "markedly reduced," and and 47.3 percent "reduced" Type A behavior. The remaining 21 percent were unaffected measurably. A significant, though smaller, percentage of patients receiving only cardiologic counseling displayed a "markedly reduced" (7.2 percent) or "reduced" (41.7 percent) Type A pattern over the course of the study, suggesting either that (1) the infarction itself modified behavior, (2) traditional counseling inadvertantly resulted in dimunition of the pattern, or (3) personal physicians or other external influences altered behavior. Those patients who changed most rapidly—that is, after the first year—had one-fourth the recurrence rate of heart attacks of those who did not. Of these, 90.6 percent were in the special counseling group. The cumulative recurrence rate of infarctions in those who actually completed the three-year study was significantly less in the Type A special counseling group (8.9 percent) than in the traditional group (18.9 percent) and in the third "comparison" group (17.1 percent). When all patients from both groups were included whether or not they actually completed the study, significant differences (7.2 percent versus 13.2 percent) remained. All of these differences were in the recurrence of *nonfatal* infarctions; there were no significant differences in mortality. These differences were not due to alterations of other risk factors.

Thus it *can* be done—and it *does* matter. In the final two chapters, we involve ourselves extensively in just how one could go about this without recourse to special counseling.

We have mentioned the reticence of some cardiologists to accept evidence implicating the TABP as a significant risk factor in coronary heart disease. This reticence continues, and is typified by a recent study purporting to demonstrate "no relation between Type A behavior and the long-term outcome of acute myocardial infarction."[19]

The study administered the Jenkins Activity Surgery to 516 patients *one to two weeks following* an acute myocardial infarction, and compared the survival of A's and B's over one to three years. There were no differences. Why should there be? Other risk factors were not measured (or at least not reported), no modifications were undertaken, and presumably all of the patients had disease of relatively similar severity. Once the disease is established, it will continue to progress for all of the reasons that resulted in its occurrence in the first place. Why should a Type A individual progress any more rapidly than a patient with hypercholesterolemia or a smoker? The fact that Type A's do not tells us little that we did not already know; namely, that the TABP is no stronger than other risks in creating or worsening coronary heart disease, and it certainly is not protective. The study makes little sense to me, yet it was a leading article in the *New England Journal of Medicine*, and its above-quoted conclusions serve only to obscure rather than clarify the impact of the TABP on coronary heart disease. Many physicians continue to resist the importance of the Type A concept.

Fear is a potent force for change. Sometimes, in the course of my practice, it has appeared to me to be the only effective motivator. Risk factor modification—by cessation of smoking,[20] reduction of cholesterol by diet or medication if necessary,[21] treatment of hypertension, abandonment of a sedentary life-style, and modification of the TABP—offers the only known hope of staving off coronary disease, or altering its course. Mr. A, and some patients like him, may survive to reevaluate their priorities and modify their risks. Far too many are not so fortunate. The information presented in this chapter suggests that such modifications are worth the time, energy, and inconvenience that they may engender. It seems logical that the

123

earlier the changes are made, the less likely the disease will occur in the first place. And as we shall see in the concluding two chapters of this book, they need not be painful, but can add dimensions of fulfillment and enjoyment to life unconceived of by the many hurried Type A's who speed their way through an already too short existence that they may, by their behavior, abbreviate even further.

REFERENCES

1. Veteran's Administration Cooperative Study Group on Hypertensive Agents. Effects of treatment on morbidity in hypertension: Results in patients with diastolic blood pressures averaging 115–129 mmHg. ,2JAMA, 202:1028–1034, 1967.
2. Veteran's Administration Cooperative Study Group on Hypertensive Agents. II. Effects of treatment on morbidity in hypertension: Results in patients with diastolic blood pressures averaging 90–114 mmHg. *JAMA*, 213:2243–1152, 1970.
3. Gifford, R. W., et al. The dilemma of mild hypertension: Another viewpoint of treatment. *JAMA*, 250:3171–3173, 1983.
4. Folsom, A. R., Luepker, R. V., Gillum, R. F., et al. Improvement in hypertension detection and control from 1973-74 to 1980-81: The Minnesota Heart Survey experience. *JAMA*, 250:916–921, 1983.
5. Kaplan, N. M. Therapy for mild hypertension. *JAMA*, 249:365–367, 1983.
6. Leonard, A. R., Igra, A., and Hawthorne, A. Status of high blood pressure control in California: A preliminary report of a statewide survey. *Heart, Lung*, 10:255, 1981.
7. Hypertension Detection and Follow-up Program Cooperative Study Group. Five-year findings of the Hypertension Detection and Follow-up Program. I. Reduction in mortality of persons with high blood pressure, including mild hypertension. *JAMA*, 242:2562–2571, 1979.
8. Australian Therapeutic Trial in Mild Hypertension. Report by the Management Committee. *Lancet*, 1:1261–1267, 1980.
9. Multiple Risk Factor Intervention Trial Research Group. Multiple risk factor intervention trial: Risk factor changes and mortality results. *JAMA*, 248:1465–1477, 1982.
10. Holland, O. B., Nixon, J. V., and Kuhnert, L. Diuretic-induced ventricular ectopic activity. *A J Med*, 70:762–768, 1981.
11. Johansson, B. W. Electrolytes and cardiac arrythmias. *Acta Med Scand Suppl*, 647:1–171, 1980.
12. Struthers, A., Whitesmith, R., and Reid, J. Prior thiazide diuretic treatment increases adrenaline-induced hypokalemia. *Lancet*, 1:1358–1360, 1983.
13. Ram, sC. V. S. Should mild hypertension be treated? *Ann Intern Med*, 99:403–405, 1983.
14. Devereux, R. B., Pickering, T. G., Harshfield, G. A., et al. Left ventricular hypertrophy in patients with hypertension: Importance of blood pressure response to regularly recurring stress. *Circulation*, 68:470–476, 1983.
15. Roskies, E., Spevack, M., Surkis, A., et al. Changing the coronary-prone

(Type A) behavior pattern in a nonclinical population. *J Behav Med*, 1:201–216, 1978.
16. Roskies, E., Kearney, H., Spevack, M., et al. Generalizability and durability of treatment effects in an intervention program for coronary-prone (Type A) managers. *J Behav Med*, 2:195–206, 1979.
17. Suinn, R. M., and Bloom., L. J. Anxiety management training for pattern A behavior. *J Behav Med*, 1:25–35, 1978.
18. Friedman, M., Thoreson, C. E., Gill, J. J., et al. Alteration of Type A behavior and reduction in cardiac recurrences in postmyocardial infarction patients. *Am Heart J*, 108:237–248, 1984.
19. Case, R. B., Heller, S. S., Case, N. B., et al. Type A behavior and survival after acute myocardial infarction. *N Engl J Med*, 312:737–741, 1985.
20. Hjermann, I., Holme, I., Velve Byre, K., et al. Effect of diet and smoking on the incidence of coronary heart disease. *Lancet*, 2:1303–1310, 1981.
21. Lipids Research Clinics Program. The Lipid Research Clinics Coronary Prevention Trial Results: I and II. Reduction in incidence of coronary heart disease and the relationship of reduction in incidence of coronary heart disease to cholesterol lowering. *JAMA*, 251:351–374, 1984.

8

UMBRELLAS: MEDICINE, MOVEMENT, AND MEDITATION

*P*erhaps you are convinced. Being a hyperreactor is detrimental to your health, or the health of your patients and you would like to do something about it. That may not be easy, in the sense that both behavioral and perceptual changes may be necessary, and these do not come quickly or effortlessly. But how does one diagnose the individual at risk, the Type A, labile hypertensive, or silent hot reactor? The Jenkins Activity Survey is not available at the corner drugstore, and the number of individuals nationwide trained to administer the Structured Interview is in the hundreds at most. These tests are research tools, and not in widespread clinical use. Fortunately for those who wish to know, patient's perceptions of themselves as A or B are likely to be quite accurate, if they exert a bit of self honesty.

In the last chapter, we discussed a study that utilized self-referral in recruiting patients for a Type A behavior modification program, and noted that 87 percent of the applicants who considered themselves "A" were judged to be so by the researchers. This was studied more rigorously in a work entitled "Self Ratings of Type A (Coronary Prone) Adults: Do Type A's Know They Are Type A's?"[1] It would seem that they do. By asking a population of 378 white male aerospace workers to check words in a list that best applied to them and comparing this with their Structured Interview results, it was found that there was "a significant linear relationship between self-ratings of Type A characteristics and interview-based

127

Type A classification." That is, the more "A" they rated themselves, the more "A" the Structured Interview rated them. Of interest was the finding that the A's tended to ignore negative aspects of the trait, such as hostility, irritability, and bossiness, and to focus on "socially acceptable" terms, such as assertiveness, outspokenness, strength, and dominance. Type A's rejected, and B's endorsed, such terms as calm, quiet, cautious, silent, and easy-going.

Let us recall that the Jenkins Activity Survey is also a self-assessment questionnaire but is designed to approach issues somewhat more subtly by evoking responses to such situations as waiting in lines or traffic jams. It ultimately relies, however, on the individual's self-perceptions.

If, after reading the foregoing chapters, you personally believe that you are Type A, you probably are. In the course of evaluating patients, your assessment coupled with their own will probably be quite accurate as to the presence of the global Type A pattern and its components.

A strong family history of hypertension, or elevated readings, though perhaps only on occasion, may represent labile or fixed hypertension.

An individual whose hands get cold, heart pounds, and is inwardly aroused by minor stressors despite outward calm, may be a silent hot reactor. This is the hardest group to define clearly, and diagnostic studies for this condition are restricted a few research facilities. Therefore, such individuals must rely, more than the other groups, on self-assessment.

Even in the setting of established coronary disease, none of the forthcoming interventions are inappropriate; I consider them of significant thereaputic value when undertaken after appropriate medical assessment.

A common response of Type A individuals to the concept of cardiovascular arousal is, "I don't *feel* aroused." In most of the studies discussed in Chapter 5 that examined the issue, there was either no association between cardiovascular reactivity and perceptions of anxiety or arousal[2,3] or *less* arousal reported by A's than B's.[4] This may be the result of long-standing adaptation to the subjective sensations of arousal, or perhaps a certain enjoyment of the aroused state (so-called adrenaline high). In any case, absence of subjective sensations, at least in A's, does not preclude frequent

UMBRELLAS: MEDICINE, MOVEMENT, AND MEDITATION

and ongoing cardiovascular hyperreactivity.

So most of us know who we are. Let us see what we, as health care providers or patients, can do about it.

If sympathomedullary arousal to psychosocial stress is a presumed mechanism of risk for coronary heart disease, and we agree that this is likely, than sympathomedullary blockade would be a logical therapeutic approach. In theory, however, such an approach could deprive us of fight-or-flight capabilities should we actually require them to cope with physical danger. Though the need for arousal is rare, its absence could be critical. In addition, those of us who exercise or enjoy challenging sports would conceivably find our capabilities to perform blunted by such blockade. Let us examine this approach, as drugs that block portions of the sympathetic nervous system are already in widespread use as a treatment for hypertension and angina.

Recall from Chapter 2 the many functions governed by the sympathetic nervous system. Also recall that this system is divided into alpha and beta components, with alpha concerned primarily with vascular tone and beta with heart rate, force of contraction, blood flow to skeletal muscle, dilatation of the airways, etc. There are alpha and beta receptors at the ends of sympathetic nerves where they interface with the target organ, whether it is arterial musculature, the heart, or the airway. These receptors respond to the presence of norepinephrine and epinephrine, and the stimulation or suppression of the target organ results.

Pharmacologic blockade of these receptors is possible through drugs that substitute for epinephrine or norepinephrine at receptor sites, but block rather than activate the receptor (Figure 14). It is possible to design drugs that selectively block the alpha or beta receptors, and such drugs have been engineered to block only certain beta receptors, termed beta-1 or beta-2. Beta-1 receptors are found primarily on the heart, whereas beta-2 receptors comprise the rest of the beta system, and thus beta-1 blocking drugs are termed "cardioselective."

Certainly if hypertension begins in some people with cardiac hyperreactivity, the so-called hyperdynamic state, then blocking that reactivity makes sense. Indeed many physicians consider beta-blockers the initial drug of choice in the young hypertensive. Until recently, such utility frequently was marred by unacceptable side effects of nonselective beta-blockade, such as somnolence and impotence; however, beta-1 blockers are now available that are much better tolerated, and also penetrate less well into brain tissue, where most of these side effects originate. Compliance with any medical regimen is critical for it to have efficacy, and silent, symptom-free hypertension is hard for the young patient to reconcile with a therapy that makes him or her feel worse than the illness.

Beta-blockers are highly effective in the treatment of hypertension. They are also used to control angina in patients with coronary heart disease, because of their depressive effect on the rate and force of cardiac contraction. This results in less work for the heart and a subsequent decrease in oxygen demand, and hence less need for blood flow through narrowed arteries. Clearly their use is limited, and is contraindicated in patients whose heart function is already marginal because of previous severe heart attacks and consequent significant muscle destruction; if given, the lungs can fill with fluid, a condition known as congestive heart failure.

There is a current controversy amoung cardiologists about the efficacy of beta-blockers in preventing further heart attacks in patients with a previous myocardial infarction. Two large, controlled studies on the impact of selective beta-blockade on mortality in the months to years following a myocardial infarction have demon-

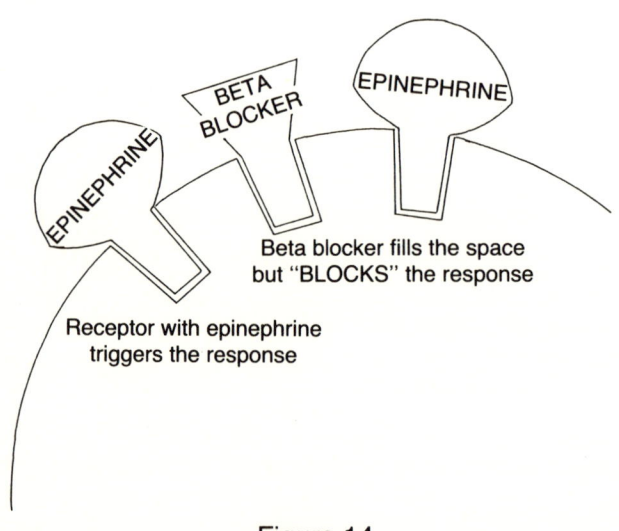

Figure 14

strated marked reduction of mortality in patients treated with these drugs.[5,6] The mechanisms are unclear, but in one study[6] the incidence of sudden death was reduced by 44 percent in the treated group. We are left with the distinct possibility that reduction in cardiovascular hyperreactivity by these agents resulted in protection from ventricular fibrillation. How many patients died in the manner described in Chapter 6, around the time of major psychological stress, is unknown. Another effect of beta-blockers that may enhance their ability to protect against recurrent infarction is that they reduce platelet adhesiveness, and so perhaps the tendency to propagate clots on arterial plaques.[7]

But are beta-blockers a reasonable therapy for cardiovascular reactivity in the Type A without clinical heart disease? Can a drug make A's into B's, physiologically or otherwise? Are the consequences of sympathetic blockade worth the benefits? Are some of our younger beta-blocked hypertensives losing more by sacrificing fight-or-flight capabilities than they gain? Let us see.

Two studies have looked at the impact of beta-blockade on the physiologic and behavioral characteristics of Type A individuals. The first employed a selective beta-blocker versus a diuretic (so-called water pill that decreases vascular volume) in 19 mildly hypertensive males classified as Type A or B by the Structured Interview. This study demonstrated a diminution in Type A characteristics in the beta-blocker group after four to ten weeks of treatment. In this group five patients shifted toward Type B as compared with the diuretic group, in which none moved in this direction, but in which four actually became more intensely "A." Speech stylistics such as loud, explosive, rapid, and accelerated, were significantly diminished in the beta-blocked group. When studied for reactivity using the Structured Interview as a stressor, regardless of A or B status, beta-blocker-treated patients were less reactive than their diuretic-treated counterparts.[8]

A second, larger study[9] involved a group of 88 patients of both sexes who already were being treated either with a nonselective beta-blocker, propranolol, or one of a number of other antihypertensive agents, none of which were beta-blockers. As all had been referred for cardiac catheterization, all had presumed coronary heart disease. This study simply compared the 65 patients under propranolol therapy with 23 not taking the drug in terms of degree of

Type A behavior, cardiovascular reactivity to stress, and severity of coronary heart disease. Again it appeared that patients medicated with a beta-blocker demonstrated less intense Type A behavior, even when other factors were controlled for. The authors point out, however, that the study was correlational, and that there were no data on Type A status prior to initiation of the drug. Patients taking this drug were less reactive, regardless of their A/B status.

How might this be? Is the A behavior altered by some effect of the drug on the brain, as with a tranquilizer? If the drugs were exerting some effect via the brain, they would depress sympathetic stimuli originating there, thereby inhibiting norepinephrine release from nerve terminals and epinephrine secretion by the adrenal medulla. One thus would expect to see lower levels of catecholamines in response to stressors in individuals medicated with beta-blockers as compared with unblocked controls. However, two studies[10,11] have demonstrated an *increase* in catecholamine levels under both physical and psychogenic stress with these drugs, implying that the stimulus from the brain for sympathetic stimulation continues, and is even enhanced. This enhancement would likely result from failure of a feedback loop to be "satisfied" that sympathetic activation had occurred.

There are, for instance, receptors in certain blood vessels and in the kidney that are stimulated by increases or decreases in blood pressure. If blood pressure falls, a signal is sent to the brain stem that results in an outflow of sympathetic impulses, an increase in heart rate, blood vessel constriction, and retention of salt by the kidney, all homeostatic changes designed to increase blood pressure. This would be a sensible response, say, to bleeding, which lowers the blood pressure. If the pressure rises, inhibitory messages are sent. If homeostasis is stressed beyond its ability to respond (by for instance, a drop in pressure approaching shock range), the stress response is stimulated, and sympathetic activation intensifies, accompanied by adrenal medullary arousal. This intensifies the homeostatic alterations and stimulates emergency mechanisms to raise pressure—that is, shunting of blood to vital organs only, an intense cardiac stimulus, etc. In the presence of beta-blockade, the receptors, being already occupied, are not stimulated by epi/norepinephrine. The rise in pressure is prevented by beta-blockade; the intensity of firing increases because the pressure does not rise and more sympathetic stimulation occurs, raising norepinephrine and epinephrine blood levels still further. It is possible to overwhelm beta-blockade by intense sympathetic stimulus. This is a saving grace, for in times of great physiologic stress, the system is still functional (dependent in part on the dose of beta-blocker being administered). It thus would appear that beta-blockers do not affect the outpouring of sympathetic stimuli by the central nervous system (see Figure 15).

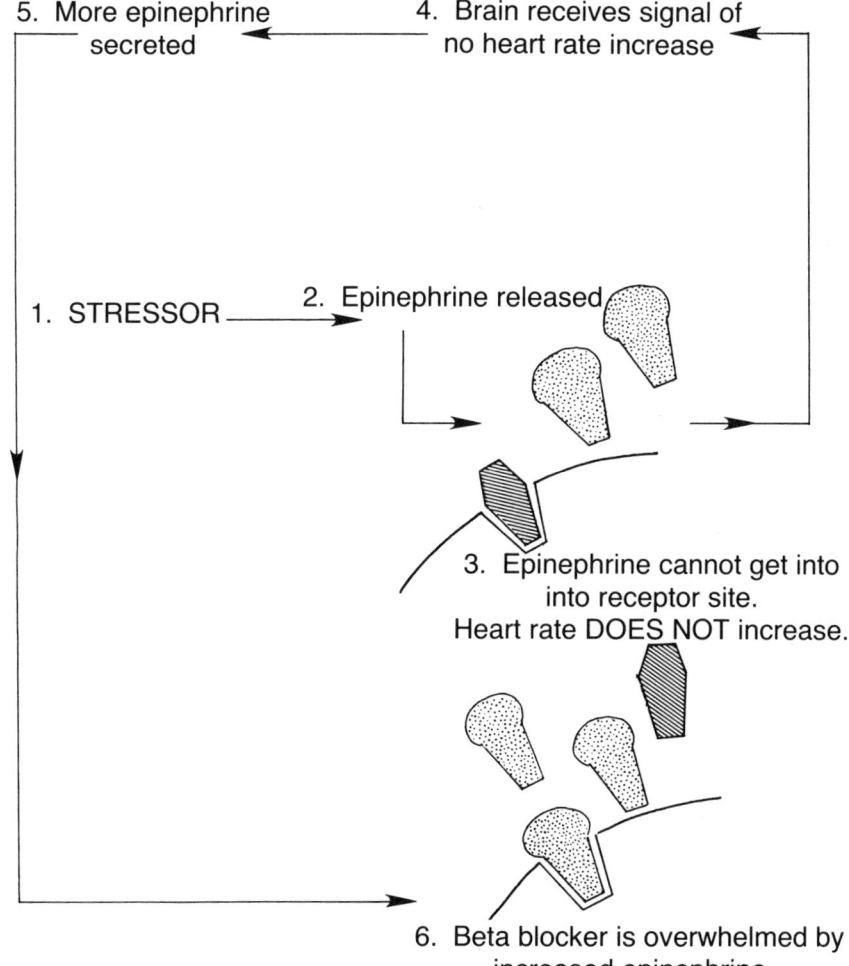

Figure 15

The drugs, then, are not sympathetic "tranquilizers."

Furthermore, certain beta-blockers have difficulty entering brain tissue because of their solubility characteristics. Yet they are just as effective in blunting sympathetic arousal, and apparently altering the Type A behavior pattern (TABP), thus suggesting that they do not affect the brain directly.[9]

Just how beta-blockers might "cool" Type A behavior is unclear, but it has been suggested that they may do so, at least in part, by eliminating anxiety-producing symptoms of arousal, such as palpitations or tremor, and breaking a cycle of anxiety begetting arousal begetting further anxiety. This receives support from studies that demonstrated marked diminution in stage fright and improvement in technical performance on the part of musicians administered these drugs.[11,12] However, anxiety is not a component of Type A behavior, although this does not rule out a "subconscious" mechanism. Another explanation might be that the Type A pattern is a behavioral *manifestation* of cardiovascular arousal, as we discussed, rather than the arousal being a physiologic accompaniment of the TABP. This is a cart/horse analogy, with physiologic arousal to psychosocial stressors the horse and TABP the cart. By slowing the horse, we slow the cart. The alteration of sympathetic arousal induced by these drugs now seemingly linked to an alteration of the behavior suggests that the two are inseparable, and that by altering one, we seem to affect the other.

Before we accept such a premise completely, let us note a caution expressed by one of the above researchers: "We should note that there was still a large preponderance of Type A patients among those who were taking propranolol. This implies that any effects of the drug were to temper somewhat the intensity of Pattern A rather than to change Type A's into B's."[9]

It might seem from these data that beta-blockade would be a reasonable therapeutic modality for Type A's in particular, and cardiovascular hyperreactors in general. Let us look at the alternative hypothesis.

Beta-blockers have been extensively studied to assess their impact on blood pressure elevation in response to both mental stress and exercise. The two studies of Type A modification by beta-blockade discussed above[8,9] demonstrated a blunted response to the Structured Interview and a history quiz in beta-blocked individuals for heart rate and blood pressure[8] and for heart rate alone.[9] Other studies in hypertensives, however, have demonstrated little ability of beta-blockers to diminish the blood pressure response to various mental stressors.[13,14] This is not surprising, if one recalls that vascular tone is mediated by alpha receptors. Stimulation of these receptors by norepinephrine raises the blood pressure by constricting the blood vessels. The heart is beta-blocked and unresponsive, but the pressure will rise simply because of an increase in the vascular resistance.

Dynamic physical exercise, on the other hand, depends on an increase in the rate and force of cardiac contraction in elevating blood pressure. Blood flow to skeletal muscle is increased, and even if there is an increase in vascular tone elsewhere, the balance between the beta-induced dilation of skeletal muscle arteries and other alpha-constricted vessels results in an overall drop or no change in vascular resistance during exercise. It is the heart that maintains the elevated pressure. With beta-blockade the heart is less able to respond to the increased demands of exercise and blood pressure elevations are attenuated. Several studies have demonstrated this.[13,15,16]

What we are left with, then, is that beta-blockers are variably effective in blunting sympathomedullary arousal in A's and hypertensives in response to psychogenic stressors, depending on whom you read; more effective in preventing heart rate and blood pressure elevations in response to dynamic physical exercise; and effective in reducing anxiety and the peripheral manifestations of arousal prior to public performance.

The impact of beta-blockers on the fight-or-flight response seems to occur notably when physical activity, especially such dynamic physical activity as running, is involved. This is apparent in the ability of beta-blockers to inhibit or markedly attenuate the conditioning effects of exercise, above and beyond their capability to blunt blood pressure and heart rate responses. This is certainly undesirable for those who wish to improve their level of fitness. A host of studies has looked at the issue in one of two ways: patients treated with beta-blockers are compared with controls in terms of improvement of exercise tolerance following a conditioning program, or the individuals are used as their own controls and tolerance compared before and after treatment. Some studies combine both formats.[17] Current knowledge of this subject may be summarized as follows:

1. Beta-blockade does seem to depress conditioning in most (but not all) studies.[17-19]
2. Nonselective blockade appears to produce more fatigue, and perhaps more of an impact on conditioning, than selective medications.[18]
3. Patients with established coronary disease demonstrate less attentuation of the training effect than normals.[20]
4. Effects are at least somewhat dose dependent.[17]

Beta-blockers are not "magic bullets" for cardiovascular hyperreactivity. They appear to interfere with physical prowess and conditioning, and are not definitively effective in preventing hyperreactivity to psychogenic stressors. They are, however, effective, well-tolerated agents for therapy in hypertension and angina, and are probably useful in preventing recurrent heart attacks. They do not totally block conditioning effects, and hence are not contraindicated in exercising individuals without coronary disease, but other alternatives may be desirable. They cannot be recommended for treatmenty of the TABP, however, except perhaps in extreme cases; they are not benign or free of adverse reactions, there are insufficient data as to their utility in this condition, and there are alternatives, as we shall see.

More important than any potential use of these drugs to depress expression of the TABP is what such an effect may teach us about the pattern; namely, that by altering sympathetic arousal, the behavioral manifestations of the pattern may follow suit.

A brief comment about drug treatment of hypertension and exercise: Alpha-blocking agents are available that decrease blood pressure by reducing vascular tone, and hence resistance; these drugs appear to depress exercise tolerance less than beta-blockade, probably because the heart is unaffected by them.[21] There are also agents that decrease the discharge of sympathetic impulses in the brain itself (called central alpha agonists) used for the treatment of hypertension; they are not considered agents of first choice because of their side effects. Interestingly, most contemporary drugs used for the treatment of hypertension depend primarily on blocking components of the sympathetic nervous system. We know enough physiology now to suspect that most hypertension must have a strong sympathetic component, which certainly is responsive to psychogenic stress. This is a stiff argument to counter for those who maintain that stress plays little role in the pathogenesis of this disorder.

One more point should be made. A common first drug of choice for the treatment of hypertension is the diuretic. But many diuretics deplete the body of potassium, thus necessitating its daily replacement. If the potassium falls, the heart becomes more vulnerable to dangerous arrythmias. In addition, many diuretics increase the serum cholesterol as well. I avoid these agents in young, active hypertensives.

Drugs, therefore, are not the answer for the normotensive Type A hyperreactor. They may not be the initial therapy of best choice for the hypertensive either, if the individual is motivated to pursue other alernatives. Let us see what else we can do.

Exercise has been touted since ancient times as a helpful tool in maintaining and recovering health. Dr. Arthur S. Leon quotes Moses Miamonides, the great 12th century Hebrew scholar and physician: "Anyone who sits around idle and takes no exercise will be subject to physical discomfort and ailing strength."[22]

Exercise is not the panacea claimed by some, but there is evidence that an active physical life, whether at work or leisure, can help to stave off clinical manifestations of CHD, if not the atherosclerotic process itself. Studies spanning four decades that have examined this premise have looked at sedentary versus active populations all over the world, and compared their relative incidence of fatal and nonfatal coronary heart disease, variously controlling for other risk factors. With the assistance of a review of the subject by Dr. Arthur S. Leon,[22] we present an overview of this literature.

The first major study of this type, performed more than 30 years ago, compared incidence of coronary heart disease in sedentary British bus drivers, postal clerks, and government civil servants with a group of London conductors on double-decker buses and ambulating or cycling postmen. There was a significantly lower incidence of coronary disease events and sudden death in the more active group, and the conductors followed through middle age had half the incidence of coronary heart disease death of the drivers.[23]

Though this study has been criticized because the drivers may have been more obese and have had higher blood pressures at the commencement of the research, the statistic has withstood the test of time in later studies reviewed by Leon; most of these found one-third to three-fourths the incidence of coronary heart disease among physically active as compared with inactive workers. As Leon points out, the few studies not in agreement with this finding displayed a lack of concordance between the job title used to make the assessment of sedentary state and the actual degree of physical work involved, or the more active group had higher levels of other risk factors that may have negated effects of exercise.[22]

A rather convincing study performed in Israel compared residents of kibbutzim (collective farms), again by their level of work-related activity and their incidence of coronary disease.[24] In addition to the relatively large numbers involved (some 10,500 men and women), the communal kitchens and ethnic homogeneity served to control in part for other risk factors. Sedentary work imposed a 2.5 times CHD risk for men and 3.1 risk for women, similar to classical risk factors and the TABP.

Leisure exercise is just as protective, it would seem, as indicated by two large studies. One followed 18,000 British civil servants for eight and a half years, and found that vigorous leisure-time activities appeared to reduce the rate of myocardial infarctions by half and death from coronary heart disease by one-third in the active versus the sedentary group. Additionally, as the population aged, the incidence of coronary heart disease increased only in the sedentary group.[25] The other large study found that among 17,000 male Harvard alumni, some of whom had been followed since 1916, active leisure pursuits again seemed capable of reducing coronary heart risks by as much as 64 percent if the level of such activity exceeded 2000 kcal/week, roughly the equivalent of four hours of aerobic exercise.[26] Ex-college athletes who became sedentary had the highest risk of all.

What is particularly telling about this study is that exercise seemed to counter, at least in part, the presence of other risk factors, particularly smoking, hypertension, and family history of coronary heart disease. The protection was not absolute, but reduced the relative risks of these other factors significantly. An element of this reduction relative to those with a family history of hypertension is that such a history in sedentary individuals was a significant risk for coronary heart disease, but not at all for the active population.[27]

Large studies of populations from around the world, including the Framingham and the Western Collaborative Group Study (WCGS) discussed in Chapter 3, have yielded contradictory results. Overall incidence of coronary heart disease was not or was only weakly associated with sedentary life-style in some, and clearly and strongly associated with it in others. Confounding variables included strong associations, in some countries, of cigarette smoking with active leisure pursuits, variable follow-up periods, methodology used to assess level of activity (i.e., reports from surviving spouses, questionnaires, job titles, etc.), and the actual end point the study measured (i.e., death, angina, myocardial infarctions, etc.). (See reference 22.)

One study, for instance, reported data from a giant cohort of individuals in seven industrialized nations, and demonstrated that, in all but three, classical risk factor prevalence better explained CHD incidence than activity.[28] However, reevaluation of the data in one of these countries with an intensive attempt to quantify activity levels caused researchers to revise the findings of the previous work, and allowed them to demonstrate an increased incidence of coronary heart disease among sedentary males in their 50s and 60s.[29]

Other, more recent population studies have found relative risks of sedentary existence varying from 1.5 in men and 2.4 in women in Finland to 1.3 for men and none for women in Framingham, Mass., to no added risk in the WCGS except in men over 50 (see reference 22).

This is a brief summary of extensive population-based research in this area, with its attendent problems and multiple variables, and is but one piece of the quilt. A different patch is autopsy evidence, which had investigated the same question under somewhat different means. I will quote the essence of these studies from Dr. Leon's review:

> 1) Autopsy evidence of death from coronary heart disease was twice as frequent in men doing light work as compared with men doing heavy work. In addition, sedentary men tended to die at an earlier age than active men.
>
> 2. In most studies the *frequency* [emphasis mine] of severe coronary atherosclerosis tended to be similar in sedentary, moderately active, and very active men . . .

3. The physically active men had *significantly larger* [emphasis mine] coronary artery luminal (inner diameter) areas compared with light workers. . . . In addition the active men were less likely than the inactive men to have total occlusions of major coronary arteries despite advanced atherosclerosis.

4. Physically active men had significantly less . . . healed infarcts than inactive men even in the presence of similar severe coronary atherosclerosis.

This body of evidence suggests that exercise does not necessarily interrupt the atherosclerotic process per se, but seems primarily to moderate its impact on the heart. It accomplishes this by apparent protection of the arteries from complete blockage that would result in frank MI, thus causing the arteries themselves to enlarge, and perhaps by protecting and strengthening the heart muscle itself.

Once again, we discover that models are not perfect, as intuitively correct as they may seem, as results in general in this and most other fields of scientific inquiry are not totally consistent. We are left to weigh the evidence and reach conclusions on which we must act, and we must do so as critically and objectively as possible. It is sometimes useful, as we saw in Chapter 3, to convene a body of experts to review the database and issue conclusions and recommendations on the basis of their concensus opinion. This has been done by the American Heart Association's Subcommittee on Exercise: "Evidence suggests that regular moderate, or vigorous occupational or leisure-time physical activity may protect against coronary heart disease and may improve the likelihood of survival from a heart attack."[30]

The evidence is compelling enough to this clinician that I strongly urge patients under my care to begin early and persist in this pursuit throughout life, or to undertake such a pursuit at any age after appropriate medical evaluation. How much exercise is protective and what risks are incurred we will discuss shortly, but let us first inquire as to how exercise might exert protection from coronary heart disease, and who might benfit the most. We will look at the influence of exercise on hypertension, cholesterol, and the TABP.

Despite the fact that an Australian review of some 37 studies on the impact of exercise on hypertension published in 1982 reported it was "not significantly different than the effects of placebo treatment,"[31] my own perusal of the literature suggests that, at least in certain subgroups of hypertensive patients, it may be a useful therapeutic modality. The "review" itself was not a review in the usual sense of the word, but a grouped statistical analysis of all nonpharmacologic antihypertensive therapy, so that data from many very different studies were pooled and only absolute statistics combined and analyzed. This obviously lumps quality studies with less precise works, and very different experimental designs are treated equally.

The first real look at exercise as an actual therapeutic regimen in hypertension was a 1970 trial of six months of walk–jog aerobics in sedentary middle-aged hypertensive males, many of whom were already receiving pharmacologic therapy. The study showed a dramatic decline of both diastolic and systolic pressures (11.8 and 13.5 mmHg respectively) in these men.[32] There was no long-term follow-up, nor were the results controlled for the possible effects of confounding factors such as weight loss or change in diet.

Adolescents with hypertension who underwent six months of aerobic training also had significant diminutions in their blood pressures. Twenty-five rather profoundly hypertensive children were studied; weight changes did not account for the observed blood pressure decrease. Furthermore, when retested nine months after exercise cessation, six of these patients, specifically those who had had both elevated systolic and diastolic pressures at intake, still had reduced diastolic pressures, although the other patients had returned to baseline.

Six of the 25 were "hyperkinetic"; that is, their hypertension was based on an elevated cardiac output as opposed to increased vascular resistance. These children had a diminution of their cardiac output after training, which suggests an amelioration of their abnormal hemodynamic state. The mechanisms of pressure elevations and reductions in the rest of these patients were less clear. A nonexercising control group had no significant change in blood pressures during the study period.[33]

It is important to note the fact that exercise did not completely normalize the blood pressure in these hypertensive adolescents; however, it did make significant inroads in this direction.

The most definitive recent study of exercise and hypertension involved 135 hypertensive men and women, approximately half of whom were already taking medication for this condition. It is worthwhile to look closely at the design and results of this work.[34]

All patients were asked to run two miles a day, and blood pressure measurements were instituted three months after this goal had been reached. Thirty patients dropped out, most because of muscle or joint pain.

Of the 58 patients with previously untreated hypertension who completed the study, only four had pressure decreases of 5 mmHg or less. The others had an average decrease of 17.4 systolic and 14.7 diastolic! Of the remaining patients already under treatment, 24 were actually able to discontinue all medication. Fourteen others decreased or eliminated at least one drug from their regimen. Weight change, either gain or loss, was not a factor in determining blood pressure control, a finding in agreement with two other studies.[35,36] The severity of hypertension at intake was also irrelevant to the success of exercise in achieving therapeutic efficacy. This observation is extremely important in that medical dogma often suggests that nontraditional, nonpharmacologic therapies for hypertension are only efficacious in mild disease.

Seventy-eight patients in this series have been followed for periods ranging from three to over ten years. Of these, 52 have relied on exercise alone to control their blood pressures.

This study could be criticized for lack of a matched control group, with some validity, as there is inadequate documentation of other potentially confounding variables, such as dietary alteration or work activity. Nonetheless, a large, mixed group of "garden variety" hypertensives who have responded so well to a nonpharmacologic intervention is certainly worth noting.

Exercise, then, appears to be a useful therapeutic intervention in many, if not most, hypertensives—at least as an adjunct to, and possibly in place of, drug therapy for some.

The impact of exercise on cholesterol needs to be examined in the context of the impact of different components of cholesterol on coronary risk. the cholesterol content of blood has several components that can be fractionated chemically, and levels of these components appear to represent differential risk for CHD. In fact, one component of cholesterol, the so-called HDL, or high-density lipoprotein, seems actually to be protective as its values increase.[37,38] It is on this component of cholesterol that exercise appears to exert much of its effect, as we shall see. Total and LDL (or low-density lipoprotein) cholesterol are associated with increased incidence of CHD, and these values may also be influenced by exercise.

The largest and most comprehensive study on the cholesterol/exercise interaction examined 7106 men with known elevations of their cholesterol, but without clinical coronary disease. The men were questionnaire-rated as to levels of work and leisure physical activity, and their responses were correlated with blood levels of HDL, LDL, and total cholesterol. Other factors, such as age, weight, alcohol intake, and smoking, were controlled for. Diet, however, was not, and remained a confounding variable in the results. Only HDL cholesterol was associated with level of physical activity; the more the exercise, the higher was the HDL. This, then, signified a salutory effect of exercise on another coronary risk factor, though it may have been mediated indirectly, perhaps by different dietary preferences in active people.[39]

Numerous smaller studies have examined this issue in a variety of ways, and are reviewed by Goldberg.[40] He concludes:

> An independent relationship between exercise, fitness, and the total level of cholesterol [and] HDL has been difficult to establish. The effects of training on these parameters may occur only as a consequence of alteration in body habitus, diet, smoking, or ethanol or medication use. Evidence to date suggests that persons with higher cholesterol [and] LDL as well as individuals with lower HDL levels have favorable changes in these measurements after either endurance or resistive exercise training.

Exercise is fairly antithetical to cigarette abuse, and we will say no more on the subject.

These are the classical risk factors. Does exercise have any capacity for modifying either the behavioral or physiologic components of the TABP? A priori, one might expect a Type A individual to relate to an exercise regimen in a similar fashion as to his or her job situation, or other challenge. Nonetheless, two studies have demonstrated an attentuation of Type A behavior after a short term (weeks) of exercise training. No long-term follow-up was available in either patient population, but both "severe" and moderate or mild Type A's (as judged by Jenkins Activity Survey scores) appeared to benefit from aerobic fitness training.[41,42]

One study compared 50 Type A and B men and women undergoing a ten-week aerobic training program as to changes in Jenkins Activity Survey scores. Type A's clearly became less A (but not B) whereas the B's were unaffected.[41]

The second study used a nonexercising control group of patients and did not divide groups into "A" or "B," although Jenkins Activity Survey scores were obtained. The sample size was quite small (six in each group) but exercising patients did display a diminution in magnitude of A behavior as compared with the nonexercising controls.[42]

Much more work has been done regarding the impact of exercise on cardiovascular reactivity, which, if our premise is correct, is quite germane to the mechanisms via which the TABP exerts its influence on the coronary vasculature.

Several studies have addressed this issue, generally by comparing cardiovascular arousal with psychosocial stressors in fit versus sedentary subjects; unfortunately only one simultaneously measured Type A characteristics.[43] In this study patients at varying levels of aerobic fitness were subjected to psychological stressors, and blood pressure, heart rate, norepinephrine values, and Type A status, among other (to us) less relevant variables, were measured at baseline and in response to these stressors. In subjects over 40, blood pressure response to the stressors was lower in fit versus nonfit individuals. All fit patients had lower resting heart rate. (This is a well-recognized consequence of aerobic training.) Epinephrine and norepinephrine levels were not related to fitness, but did increase in all patients in response to the stressors, indicating arousal.

There are several useful observations to be made from this work, as well as several problems with it, at least from our perspective. With regard to problems, the study compared patients who were self-selected in terms of their own fitness as opposed to persons undergoing training as part of a protocol. Patients who choose to exercise probably possess different psychological profiles than those who do not. Consequently it would be difficult to attach much significance to their A/B:fitness profiles. Moreover, since such profiles were not generated, we do not know the distribution of fit A's, sedentary B's, etc. We are unable to tell from the data whether trained A's are less aroused than their less fit counterparts or than untrained B's, and so on. Because of the self-selection design of the study, and the way the data were analyzed, we can look at the fitness effect, but can say little about its relationship to the A or B pattern, despite the fact that patients were evaluated by the Jenkins Activity Survey.

This does not detract from the work, as it does not seem that the authors were specifically addressing the A/B fitness question. What they did demonstrate was that fit subjects over 40 years of age were less reactive to psychogenic stressors than untrained individuals, despite the fact that their catecholamine levels elevated equally. This suggests a decrease in sensitivity of the peripheral catecholamine receptors in trained individuals, as opposed to a depression of catecholamine release in response to the stressor. By this we mean that when the catecholamine arrives at its target organ, its impact, or ability to stimulate that structure, is diminished by the training effect, via a mechanism or mechanisms unknown. This has essentially the same impact as a smaller amount of the neurotransmitter arriving at the target site, in that the evoked response is diminished. This is interesting because the mechanism of some antihypertensive drugs, as discussed earlier, is to block the catecholamine receptors in various tissues, without necessarily affecting catecholamine release. The important fact remains, however, that reactivity was diminished in this study by exercise.

Another perspective on this phenomenon is offered by a work that investigated autonomic *recovery* time in response to psychosocial stressors in fit versus unfit subjects, presuming that arousals during the stressor might be similar.

Furthermore, the researchers addressed the issue of self-selection by looking at previously fit individuals, at those who were voluntarily beginning to train, and at those trained as part of a randomly assigned protocol. Appropriate controls were included. They also compared exercise with meditation and music appreciation for their relative capacities to attenuate poststressor arousal duration.

Their results showed that fitness per se, self-selected or not, was associated with less arousal during stressors, and more rapid heart rate recovery following the challenge. This held true across a variety of stressors, and in comparison with meditation and music appreciation, as well. Furthermore, individuals who were untrained at baseline demonstrated definite improvement in autonomic recovery over time as their fitness improved, a phenomenon that did not occur in the other groups.[44]

Certainly such results have the capacity to benefit the hyperreactor if prolonged reactivity after the stressor has passed is instrumental in cardiovascular damage, as one might speculate.

Three other studies, not quite as complex in design, demonstrated similar findings.[45-47] An interesting observation by one of these groups, Sinyor et al.,[45] was that catecholamines rose faster, peaked sooner, and returned to baseline faster during a series of psychogenic stressors in trained versus untrained subjects. This has been interpreted as an adaptive phenomenon, representing an anticipatory response to prepare for the stressor, with rapid recovery following.

How much and what kind of exercise is necessary to exert a protective effect against coronary heart disease appears to be a minimum of one hour per day of physical labor, such as lifting, carrying, or shoveling (intermittent anaerobic) or 30 minutes per day of vigorous leisure activity, such as jogging or swimming (aerobic). Maximum jogging benefit for coronary heart disease protection appears to accrue at approximately 20 miles per week of walking or jogging for an average-sized male (see review by Leon[22]). Little is known quantitatively about the level of exercise necessary to attentuate cardiovascular hyperreactivity.

Whenever an individual dies during vigorous physical activity such as jogging it is a noteworthy, and often newsworthy, phenomenon. Autopsy studies have demonstrated that such deaths are usually the result of occult coronary disease, and occur in runners who begin later in life and who possess risk factors for coronary heart disease. Often it seems that they ignored or denied chest pains that may have represented anginal episodes prior to the fatal event. This appears to have been the case with Jim Fixx, the author whose books on the joys of running inspired many a novice jogger, including this writer. The mechanism of death appears to be an arrhythmia precipitated by the supply/demand imbalance of narrowed coronaries inadequately supporting the working heart muscle. Recall that an ischemic, or oxygen-starved, heart is more irritable and prone to such rhythm, disorders. Occasionally sudden death during exercise occurs in young, healthy athletes who at autopsy are found not to have had coronary heart disease, but instead may have suffered a hemorrhage into the brain from a congenitally weak blood vessel, may have been born with a hitherto-undiscovered cardiac defect, used cardiotoxic drugs such as cocaine, or may have suffered heat stroke. Such events are rare.[22]

Patients who have multiple risk factors, have established angina, or have sustained actual infarction can benefit from aerobic exercise training. An important part of therapy following a heart attack is cardiac rehabilitation exercise, which begins two to three days after the event, providing there are no complications. Exercise is graded, and patients generally are able to climb stairs within ten to 14 days after the event. In the weeks to months following, progressive walking and other aerobic activities are prescribed, limited by the patient's symptoms. Exercise tolerance almost invariably improves. Fatal or nonfatal cardiac events in such programs are extremely rare.[22]

The most important screening procedure for patients at risk for coronary heart disease or who have established disease is the graded exercise-tolerance or treadmill test. This allows the physician to quantitate the level of exercise that causes no electrocardiogram changes, such as ST-segment depression, and to set a safe course of exercise for the patient. Repeated testing can be motivational in that patients can see the improvement in their exercise tolerance. I have also found in my practice that many individuals who were dismayed at their initially poor physical condition became motivated to improve. These most frequently are patients with risk factors whom I try to inspire to make positive life-style changes, but who are not convinced solely by my words. The test thus serves a dual purpose.

Exercise is an active way of dealing with cardiovascular reactivity and its attendant consequences. Most of the work in the field shows that it is well worth the investment of time and energy, if for no other reason than the improvement in self-esteem that seems to attend improved fitness, although more significantly for its apparent cardioprotective effects. Exercise may have its consequences, and has been likened by some to an addiction; some aerobic athletes are undoubtedly as "A" about this as they are about work. Nonetheless exercise has few side effects and appears to exert benefit with regard to a variety of cardiovascular risk factors.

Passive behavioral methods of coping with hyperreactivity and Type A behavior have been espoused in recent years. They include meditation, biofeedback, self-hypnosis, and various "relaxation" therapies, and a spate of research has been published regarding their physiologic effects and efficacy in coping with hypertension in particular, and other risk factors in general.

What all of these techniques share is passivity in the sense that they involve sitting quietly for 20–40 minutes once or twice a day and concentrating on a word, image, feeling, or electronic signal. They also have some important differences, both in technique and efficacy.

Biofeedback is a technological method of translating physiologic phenomena into auditory or visual signals that would otherwise be undetectable to the individual in whom these phenomena are taking place. For instance, unless we are exercising or are very anxious, we are unaware of our heart rate. Similarly, unless the blood pressure is high enough to cause dramatic medical problems such as elevation of the pressure inside the brain or hemorrhage into the eyes, or low enough not to perfuse vital organs, it is essentially an asymptomatic phenomenon. Relatively recently in the Western world (yogis claim to have had this knowledge for centuries), it has been found possible consciously to alter body functions considered "involuntary," such as heart rate and blood pressure, by becoming aware of them and their minute-to-minute changes. Patients may effectively learn to lower or raise these functions, as well as muscle tension and brain-wave patterns. It is not possible to instruct an individual exactly how to do this. Rather one learns a "feeling" associated with changing the given parameter by receiving feedback on the parameter, and to reproduce the feeling associated with the desired change. In essence only the desire to create the change is conscious; the details of the method appear to be subconscious, and conscious trying interferes.

In meditation one focuses on a word, sound, or visual image while excluding other conscious thoughts as much as possible—In particular, the technique of transcendental meditation, taught the United States under the auspices of Maharishi Mahesh Yogi, has been studied rather extensively, particularly by its devotees. H. Benson, a Boston cardiologist, has "demystified" the technique, and has studied it rather thoroughly as well.[48]

Progressive relaxation, first espoused by Jacobson in 1939, involves the tensing and relaxing of muscle groups in an orderly fashion. This also requires suppression of conscious thought and concentration on the sensations taking place in the limbs.

Many of the studies on the utility of these techniques in the control of blood pressure are hampered by methodological inadequacies, such as failure to include control groups, alteration of medical regimens during the course of the study, short-term or no follow-up, and lack of standardization of methods. Nonetheless there are enough studies with enough data to warrant careful attention to these interventions.

The data on biofeedback are not consistent, and results even in the positive studies have not been impressive (see references 49 and 50). Furthermore, the instrumentation is cumbersome and expensive. Biofeedback is, however, capable of lowering blood pressure in the laboratory setting, and one recent study did demonstrate success in sustained lowering of pressure in hypertensives who continued to practice the technique at home.[53] Biofeedback has been most successful when combined with a relaxation technique.[60]

Meditation/relaxation techniches have the advantage of simplicity, portability (no equipment required), and apparently greater efficacy in blood pressure control than biofeedback. A recent review of the subject[50] concludes:

> Several well-controlled studies have been reported and replicated showing prolonged and significant changes in BP in hypertensive subjects. Studies have shown persistent beneficial effects for follow-up periods as long as a year. Importantly, these changes have generally been noted in "basal" BP readings, taken at times of the day when the particular relaxation technique was *not* being practiced.

There are several observations and refinements to add to this overall picture of an effective, passive, nonpharmacologic approach to the treatment of hypertension. Efficacy has been documented for mild to severe hypertension often additive to drug effects, but sometimes as effective as medical therapy. Several different techniques of both meditation and relaxation have demonstrated effectiveness. There are, as we have come to expect, studies that show no, or clinically insignificant, effects,[51,52] but, conversely, other studies have demonstrated reductions in pressure as great as 26 mmHg (average).[53]

A recent series of studies reported by Glascow et al.[54,55] in 90 borderline hypertensives reported significant blood pressure reductions for 18 months with relaxation therapy, biofeedback, or a combination thereof, with the last the most effective. Furthermore, 13 of 44 patients originally on antihypertensives were able to discontinue their medication and maintain reduced pressures at nine-month follow-up.

We find, therefore, that blood pressures are lowered not only during the relaxation procedure itself, but during daily activities at home, and presumably elsewhere. Further, the effects were seen to persist for as long as a year if the practice was continued,[56] and there is no reason to believe that efficacy would diminish beyond this time.

Little formal study of the impact of biofeedback/relaxation therapy on the Type A behavior pattern has been undertaken. However, harkening back to our discussion of prehypertensive individuals and their presumed cardiovascular hyperreactivity, one could speculate that relaxation techniques, which might diminish sympathetic tone (relaxation is the antithesis of the fight-or-flight response), would be more efficacious in Type A's or hot reacting hypertensives. Of 30 borderline or mild hypertensives trained in the rather time-consuming practice of progressive muscle relaxation, more than 50 percent were considered responders to the technique. These responders were characterized by elevated norepinephrine levels and faster basal heart rates, which suggests that the hyperkinetic hyperreacting labile hypertensives were successfully "cooled" by relaxation.[57]

Another study[58] found a decrease in renin and aldosterone levels concomitantly with blood pressure in patients treated with a biofeedback regimen (recall that these hormones are important in salt balance and blood pressure control, and are elevated in some labile hypertensives who have increased sympathetic tone).

These are, unfortunately, the only works I could find that deal with the impact of relaxation therapy on cardiovascular hyperreactivity. This topic would seem to be a natural for further research.

One group of researchers has investigated the impact of relaxation therapies and biofeedback on other coronary risk factors as well as blood pressure. They demonstrated "significant reduction in blood pressure in all treated groups; highly significant reduction in the number of cigarettes smoked by smokers; and reduction of [cholesterol] . . . particularly in the hypertensive group."[59] There were several methodological problems inherent in this work that render interpretation of the results difficult; for instance, smokers were volunteers who were interested in cutting down or quitting, and were given antismoking literature as well as the relaxation training, and there was no evaluation of dietary changes to explain cholesterol effects. Still, it is difficult to argue with the success of the regimen, despite the fact that we cannot attribute it solely to the biofeedback/relaxation training.

A potentially lethal criticism of all studies on these techniques is that perhaps it is not the technique itself but the expectation of success that reduces the blood pressure. This is the elusive "placebo effect," and if that were indeed the case, would imply an entirely different mechanism for pressure reduction than induction of decreased sympathetic drive by the method itself.

A rather ingenious way to examine this question was developed by Aas et al.[60] They divided 30 hypertensives into two groups, both of which were trained in a muscle-relaxation technique. The only difference was that one group was told to expect benefits immediately, while the other was told the effect would be delayed. The differences were dramatic, with the immediate group experiencing an average fall in pressure of 17 mmHg, versus 2.4 mmHg for those who expected a delayed response. Both groups were essentially matched for age, sex, and severity and duration of hypertension.

The implications of this work will occupy us for a significant portion of the final chapter of this book, as it seems that the cognitive process (conscious thought) has a tremendous impact on both health and disease states. We will soon tie Type A behavior, reactivity, hypertension, and coronary disease to that most elusive of phenomena, human awareness. We may find that we have far more conscious influence on our physical status than we know. This puts an onus of choice upon us, as we will soon discuss.

Let us leave this chapter with the conclusion that whatever the mechanisms involved (and to the practicing clinician or the patient these may be only marginally relevant), both exercise and relaxation therapies can have a significant impact on cardiovascular hyperreactivity, hypertension, other CHD risk factors, and, by implication, CHD itself. Whether one wishes to generate the motivation in one's patients to pursue these time-consuming behaviors is a personal decision; as with patients in my practice, I can only present the evidence and allow the reader to make an informed judgment. I am convinced, however, that the time and energy expended will reap significant benefits, without the side effects associated with pharmocologic approaches. There will be many instances when combined therapy is necessary and desirable, but drug dosages in these circumstances may be reduced, and other risk factors favorably affected that are not altered by medication.

This says nothing about the purely esthetic and psychological benefits one may experience with improved fitness, nor does it speak to the lower levels of anxiety reported in patients who practice passive relaxation techniques.[57,58] Certainly if we accept the premise that patients share at least some responsibility for their own health maintainence, and that the easy way—medication—is not necessarily the best, then the interventions described in this chapter are worthy of our attention.

REFERENCES

1. Herman, S., Blumenthal, J. A., Black, G. M., et al. Self ratings of Type A (coronary prone) adults: Do Type A's know they are Type A's? *Psychosom Med*, 43:405–413, 1981.
2. Dembroski, T. M. Macdougall, J. M., Shields, J. L., et al. Components of the Type A coronary-prone behavior pattern and cardiovascular responses to psychomotor performance challenge. *J Behav Med*, 1:159–175, 1978.
3. Manuck, S. B., Craft, S., and Gold, K. J. Coronary-prone behavior pattern and cardiovascular response. *Psychophysiology*, 15:403–411, 1978.
4. Malcolm, A. T., Janisse, M. P., and Dyck, D. G. Type A behavior, heart rate and pupillary response: Effects of cold pressor and ego threat. *J Psychosom Res*, 28:27–34, 1984.
5. Hjalmarson, A., Herlitz, J., Malek, I., et al. Effect on mortality of metroprolol in acute myocardial infarction. *Lancet*, 2:823–827, 1981.
6. Norwegian Multicenter Study Group. Timolol-induced reduction in mortality and reinfarction in patients surviving acute myocardial infarction. *N Engl J Med*, 304:801–807, 1981.
7. Campbell, W. B., Callahan, K. S., Johnson, A. R., et al. Anti-platelet activity of beta-adrenergic antagonists: Inhibition of thromboxane synthesis and platelet aggregation in patients receiving long-term propranolol treatment. *Lancet*, 2:1382–1384, 1981.
8. Schmieder, R., Friedrich, G., Neus, H., et al. The influence of beta blockers on cardiovascular reactivity and Type A behavior pattern in hypertensives. *Psychosom Med*, 45:417–423, 1983.
9. Krantz, D. S., Durel, L. A., Davia, J. E., et al. Propranolol medication among coronary patients: Relationship to Type A behavior and cardiovascular response. *J Hum Stress*, 12:4–12, 1982.
10. Dimsdale, J. E., Hartley, H., Ruskin, J., et al. Effect of beta blockade on

plasma catecholamine levels during psychological and exercise stress. *Am J Cardiol*, 54:182–185, 1984.
11. Taggart, P., Carruthers, M., and Somerville, W. Electrocardiogram, plasma catecholamines and lipids, and their modification by oxyprenolol when speaking before an audience. *Lancet*, 2:341–346, 1973.
12. Neftel, K. A., Adler, R. H., and Kappeli, L. Stage fright in musicians: A model illustrating the effects of beta blockers. *Psychosom Med*, 44:461–469, 1982.
13. Francois, B, Cahen, R., Gravejat, M. J., et al. Do beta blockers prevent pressor responses to mental stress and physical exercise? *Europ Heart J*, 5:348–353, 1984.
14. Heidbreder, E., Pagel, G., and Heidland, A. Beta-adrenergic blockade in stress protection. Limited effects of metropolol in psychological stress. *Europ J Clin Pharmacol.* 14:391–398, 1978.
15. Shinebourne, E., Fleming, J., and Hamer, J. Effects of beta adrenergic blockade during exercise in hypertensive and ischaemic heart disease. *Lancet*, 2:1217–1220, 1967.
16. MacFarlane, B. J., Hughson, R. L., Green, H. J., et al. Effects of oral propranolol and exercise protocol on indices of aerobic function in normal man. *Canad J Physiol Pharmacol*, 61:1010–1016, 1983.
17. Marsh, R. C., Hiatt, W. R., Brammell, H. L., et al. Attenuation of exercise conditioning by low dose beta-adrenergic blockade. *J Am Coll Cardiol*, 2:551–556, 1983.
18. McCloud, A. A., Kraus, W. E., and Williams, R. S. Effects of betal-selective and nonselective beta-adrenoreceptor blockade during exercise conditioning in healthy adults. *Am J Cardiol*, 53:1656–1661, 1984.
19. Sable, D. L., Brammell, H. L., Sheehan, M. W., et al. Attentuation of exercise conditioning by beta-adrenergic blockade. *Circulation*, 65:679–684, 1982.
20. Pratt, C. M., Welton, D. E., Squires, W. G., et al. Demonstration of training effect during chronic beta adrenergic blockade in patients with coronary disease. *Circulation*, 64:1125–1129, 1981.
21. Lund-Johnson, P. Hemodynamic changes at rest and during exercise in long-term prazosin therapy for essential hypertension. *Postgrad Med*, 45–52, Nov. 1975.
22. Leon, A. S. Physical activity levels and coronary heart disease: Analysis of epidemiologic and supporting studies. *Med Clin N Am*, 69:3–20, 1985.
23. Morris, J. N., Heady, J. A., Raffle, P. A. B., et al. Coronary heart disease and physical activity of work. *Lancet*, 2:1053–1057, 1111–1120, 1953.
24. Brunner, D., Manelis, G., Modan, M., et al. Physical activity at work and the incidence of myocardial infarction, angina pectoris and death due to ischemic heart disease: An epidemiologic study in Israeli collective settlements (kibbutzim). *J Chron Dis*, 27:217–233, 1974.
25. Chave, S. P. W., Morris, J. N., Moss, S., et al. Vigorous exercise in leisure time and the death rate: A study of male civil servants. *J Epidemiol Commun Health*, 32:239, 1978.
26. Paffenberger, R. S., Wing, A. L., and Hyde, R. T. Physical activity as an index of heart attack risk in college alumni. *am J Epidemiol*, 108:161–175, 1978.
27. Paffenberger, R. S., Hyde, R. T., Wing, A. L., et al. A natural history of athleticism and cardiovascular health. *JAMA*, 252:491–495, 1984.

28. Keys, A. *Seven Countries: A Multivariate Analysis of Death and Coronary Disease.* Cambridge, Mass.: Harvard University Press, 1980.
29. Karvonen, M. J. Physical activity in work and leisure time in relation to cardiovascular diseases. *Ann Clin Res*, 14(suppl. 34):118–123, 1982.
30. American Heart Association Subcommittee on Exercise/Cardiac Rehabilitation. Statement on exercise. *Circulation*, 64:1302–1304, 1981.
31. Andrews, G., MacMahon, S. W., et al. Hypertension: Comparison of drug and non-drug treatments. *Br Med J*, 284:1523–1526, 1982.
32. Boyer, J. L., and Kasch, F. W. Exercise therapy in hypertensive men. *JAMA*, 211:1668–1671, 1970.
33. Hagberg, J. M., Goldring, D., et al. Effect of exercise training on the blood pressure and hemodynamic features of hypertensive adolescents. *Am J Cardiol*, 52:763–768, 1983.
34. Cade, R., Mars, D., et al. Effect on aerobic exercise training on patients with systemic arterial hypertension. *Am J Med*, 77:785–790, 1984.
35. Choquette, G., and Ferguson, R. J. Blood pressure reduction in "borderline" hypertensives following physical training. *Canad Med Assoc J*, 108:699–703, 1973.
36. Krotkiewski, M., Konstantinos, M., Sjostrom, L., et al. Effect of long term physical training on body fat, metabolism, and blood pressure in obesity. *Metabolism*, 328:650–658, 1979.
37. Heiss, G., Johnson, N. J., and Reiland, S. The epidemiology of plasma high density lipoprotein cholesterol levels. *Circulation*, 62(suppl IV):116, 1980.
38. Witztum, J., and Schonfeld, G. High density lipoprotein. *Diabetes*, 28:326, 1979.
39. Gordon, D. J., Witztum, J. L., Hunninghake, D., et al. Habitual physical activity and high density lipoprotein cholesterol in men with primary hypercholesterolemia: The Lipid Research Clinics Coronary Prevention Trial. *Circulation*, 67:512–520, 1983.
40. Goldberg, L., and Elliot, D. L. The effect of physical activity on lipid and lipoprotein levels. *Med Clin N Am*, 69:41–55, 1985.
41. Blumenthal, J. A., Williams, R. S., Williams, R. B., et al. Effects of exercise on the Type A (coronary-prone) behavior pattern. *Psychosom Med*, 42:289–296, 1980.
42. Lobitz, C. W., Brammell, H. L., Stoll, S., et al. Physical exercise and anxiety management training for cardiac stress management in a nonpatient population. *J Card Rehab*, 3:683–688, 1983.
43. Hull, E. M., Young, S. H., and Ziegler, M. G. Aerobic fitness affects cardiovascular and catecholamine responses to stressors. *Psychophysiology*, 21:353–360, 1984.
44. Keller, S., and Seraganian, P. Physical fitness level and autonomic reactivity to psychosocial stress. *J Psychosom Res*, 28:279–287, 1984.
45. Sinyor, D., Schwartz, S. G., Peronnet, F., et al. Aerobic fitness level and reactivity to psychosocial stress: Physiological, biochemical, and subjective measures. *Psychosom Med*, 45:205–217, 1983.
46. Cox, J. P., Evens, J. F., and Jamieson, J. L. Aerobic power and tonic heart rate responses to psychosocial stressors. *Person Soc Psych Bull*, 5:160–163, 1979.
47. Keller, S. Physical fitness hastens recovery from emotional stress. *Med Sci Sports Exerc*, 12:118, 1980.

48. Benson, H., Rosner, B. A., Marzetta, B. R., et al. Decreased blood pressure in borderline hypertensive subjects who practiced meditation. *J Chron Dis*, 27:163–169, 1973.
49. Seer, P. Psychological control of essential hypertension: Review of the literature and methodological critique. *Psychol Bull*, 86:1015–1043, 1979.
50. Frumkin, K., Nathan, R. J., Prout, M. F., et al. Nonpharmacologic control of essential hypertension in man: A critical review of the experimental literature. *Psychosom Med*, 40:294–320, 1978.
51. Pollack, A. A., Case, D. B., Weber, M. A., et al. Limitations of Transcendental Meditation in the treatment of essential hypertension. *Lancet*, 1:71–73, 1977.
52. Frankel, B. L., Patel, D. J., Horowitz, D., et al. Treatment of hypertension with biofeedback and relaxation techniques. *Psychosom Med*, 40:276–293, 1978.
53. Patel, C., and North, W. R. S. Randomized controlled trial of yoga and biofeedback in management of hypertension. *Lancet*, 1:93–95, 1975.
54. Glascow, M. S., Gaarder, K. R., and Engel, B. T. Behavioral treatment of high blood pressure. II. Acute and sustained effects of relaxation and systolic blood pressure biofeedback. *Psychosom Med*, 44:155–170, 1982.
55. Engel, B. T., Glascow, M. S., and Gaarder, K. R. Behavioral treatment of high blood pressure. III. Followup-up results and treatment recommendations. *Psychosom Med*, 45:23–29, 1983.
56. Bali, L. R. Long-term effect of relaxation on blood pressure and anxiety levels of essential hypertensive males: A controlled study. *Psychosom Med*, 41:637–646, 1979.
57. Cottier, C., Shapiro, K., and Julius, S. Treatment of mild hypertension with progressive muscle relaxation: Predictive value of indexes of sympathetic tone. *Arch Intern Med*, 144:1954–1958, 1984.
58. Patel, C., Marmot, M. G., and Terry, D. J. Controlled trial of biofeedback-aided behavioral methods in reducing mild hypertension. *Br Med J*, 282:2005–2008, 1981.
59. Patel, C., and Carruthers, M. Coronary risk factor reduction through biofeedback-aided relaxation and meditation. *J Roy Coll Gen Pract*, 27:401–405, 1977.
60. Agras, W. S., Horne, M., and Taylor, C. B. Expectation and the blood-pressure-lowering effects of relaxation. *Psychosom Med*, 44:389–395, 1982.

9
RAINBOWS

I began this investigation on Type A behavior in an attempt to sort out truth from fancy regarding "stress" as a medical phenomenon. Much that *is* fanciful has been written on the topic in the lay literature, ranging from stress as a cause of *all* diseases to nutritional cures for stress states. Stress management workshops abound, and often emphasize one or several techniques for reducing the impact of stress on the body. I have attempted to survey the body of medical literature on this aspect of the stress phenomenon, and allow the reader to draw his or her own conclusions. I believe that rational decisions and life-style changes are possible and feasible, given adequate information and motivation. I conclude this discussion of the impact of stress on the cardiovascular system with some thoughts on the "essence of A'ness," barriers to change, and possibilities for redemption based on what I now consider to be true.

We know much about the externals and physiologic internals of Type A behavior. But what about the inner workings, the thought processes, of "A"? Can we generate any useful generalizations that may give us insight into who A's are, what they desire, what they fear? For those labile hypertensives or silent hot reactors, what conclusions are possible about thought content and reactivity?

A basic concept in these considerations is that reactivity to an event is likely to be predicated on its meaning to the individual, unless it occurs under general anaesthesia in some A's with coronary disease, as we discussed. The context (threatening, challenging, controllable, uncontrollable) is a perceptual one, based on the individual's previous experience or expectations. What we are saying, in essence, is that the activation of the stress response is dependent on the perception of the event as stressful.

It is useful, therefore, to overview the process of assessment prompted by confrontation with a stressor, and to look at how A's and others might preferentially exploit certain appraisal and coping methodologies, in order to explain how they might perceive environmental events and their physiologic responses to them.

When confronted with a stressor, according to Folkman,[1] the first order of business by A's and others is the *primary appraisal*. Here an event is rapidly assessed as irrelevant, benign, or stressful. If the last, the event is further evaluated for its dimensions of challenge, threat, or, of greatest potency, harm/loss. This assessment is based on belief systems, past experience, and one's values or commitments.

A particularly important dimension in both the primary and subsequent appraisals of a stressor is that of *controllability*. This refers to the individual's belief as to whether he or she can influence the event or its impact. This may be somewhat situation independent in the sense that there appear to be two reasonably distinct modes of assessing this parameter: internal and external locus-of-control paradigms.[2] Those who are internal locus perceivers tend to view most environmental circumstances as amenable to their control, whereas external locus copers tend to perceive events as a product of fate, divinity, or other, more powerful humans. Most people utilize both techniques to some degree, but tend to demonstrate a marked preference for one or the other. Not surprisingly, Type A's generally are internal locus types, and place great value on this fact.

After primary appraisal the stressor is evaluated as to alternatives for response, a process termed secondary appraisal. Here the demands of the situation are considered in light of available coping resources, and a course of action selected or an emotional commitment made. This is called *coping*.

Coping is defined by Folkman as: "Cognitive and behavioral efforts to master, reduce, or tolerate the internal and/or external demands that are created by the stressful transaction." Within this context have been defined two relatively discrete functions of the coping process: regulation of emotions (emotion focused) and dealing with the issue itself (problem focused). *Effectiveness* is irrelevant to these definitions.

Emotion-focused coping attempts to deal with the meaning or importance of the event. Folkman relates such reactions as "Oh, it doesn't matter much," "It could have been worse," or "I'm a stronger person for having gone through this" as examples of this coping mechanism. Here one defuses the significance of the event, particularly in circumstances where it is deemed uncontrollable.

Problem-focused coping involves concrete plans of action, or "strategies." This is a very "A" technique, but certainly not limited to A's alone. It implies a sense of control, that something can be done actively to alter the situation. This coping mechanism is more common, as we would expect, among internal locus individuals, who tend to exploit cognitive alternatives more than emotional filtering.

Most coping involves a combination of the two types, but individuals tend to prefer to use one or the other for most stressors.

Two other coping modalities bear mentioning. *Suppression* is a technique wherein a conscious decision is made not to think about or dwell upon a situation even though the realities are not ignored. This is frequently employed when an event is perceived as uncontrollable by an internal locus individual, and it has become apparent that dwelling on the situation will not be fruitful, but is leading to emotional discomfort. It might be considered a mixed emotion- and problem-focused approach.

Denial, conversely, involves a refusal to admit that the stressor exists, even to oneself, and might be termed an unconscious emotion-focused coping technique.

Type A's in one study previously discussed[3] were found to employ suppression more than B's in response both to threat to self-esteem and to threat of shock, with more denial in the face of threat to self-esteem. We might recall that the A's in this study were more physiologically aroused than the B's, the implication being that neither of these coping tools is effective in diminishing hyperreactivity.

Clearly, at some point certain situations must be labeled uncontrollable, either because they are overwhelming or because active response options are limited or nonexistent. At that point a third option, *secondary control*,[4] may be exercised. In this coping modality, one may assume the attitude that "this is meant to be for my greater good," or "go with the flow and take it day to day." This would be a type of emotion-focused coping in which control is relinquished, perhaps to a higher authority, and one that involves some degree of suppression.

Initially it would seem that the problem-focused approach would be the most useful stress-reducing coping tool available, and in controllable circumstances this may be true. It enables logical, direct approaches to a problem, allowing one either to alter circumstances or to remove oneself from them. However, an internal locus individual who assumes an event is controllable when it is not may enhance the impact of the stressor by fruitless striving and subsequent frustration. One would suspect this would be particularly hard on Type A's.

All of the above could be summarized in the time-honored, if somewhat worn, "God give me the strength to change the things I can change, the courage to accept the things I cannot change, and the wisdom to know the difference." Another way to say this might be, "You got to know when to hold 'em, and know when to fold 'em."

What are the reactivity correlates of the various coping strategies? Active effortful coping *is* associated with heart rate and blood pressure elevations according to several studies.[5,6] We would expect this to be so, based on a presumed evolutionary advantage of sympathetic arousal preceding challenge, which has been primarily physical for most of our geneologic existence. Perhaps it continues to be helpful in the face of psychogenic challenge, although, as we have discussed, laboratory studies have suggested otherwise. We do know that A's tend to exert greater effort than B's to master environmentally threatening conditions, with attendant physiologic reactivity.

There is information to suggest that Type A's set very high standards for achievement, and when they are unable to meet these standards, tend to blame themselves and attribute failure to internal shortcomings. B's, conversely, perceive failure as due to external forces such as luck or providence.[7]

What is apparent from the foregoing is that A's are problem-focused, internal-locus-of-control copers. Some A's appear to set high, ambiguous standards for success and perceive failure as a threat to self-esteem, which is associated with sympathomedullary arousal, a stress response. This leads us to generate a hypothesis: Certain Type A individuals have difficulty in relinquishing their concepts of controllability in the face of failure. They are unable to employ emotion-focused coping except for denial and/or suppression. As a consequence they do not defuse the meaning or importance of the stressor to themselves, but strive harder in the face of an apparently insurmountable situation. As a result they face ongoing physiologic hyperreactivity.

I find validity in this conceptualization as a result of much of the information we have examined. Perhaps this is the basis of the A's success in the business and professional world—striving against seemingly insurmountable odds, driven by an internal goad to do and to achieve more and more. Our folklore and music are full of such ideas: "to dream the impossible dream," "to never say die," "when the going gets tough, the tough get going." Much human success must be attributable to such determination and perseverance, and the perception of uncontrollability is surely relative to some degree to the amount of effort one is willing to exert. Therefore, the key must lie in two dimensions of perception: (1) a determination of the relative importance of the object to be gained, the hurdle to be overcome, etc., and (2) a realistic appraisal of the congruity between one's capabilities and that goal. Obviously the more critical the goal (survival), the harder one would strive to attain it. It is upon such appraisals that the utility of sympathomedullary arousal must rest. Surely, in a survival situation, active coping maneuvers enhanced by adrenalin have had a tremendous evolutionary advantage. Conversely, increasing productivity of widgets may enhance one's fiscal fitness, but at the cost of the consequences of chronic reactivity to nonphysical challenge. And it is not that A's are necessarily more *effective* at what they do, but that they are probably more *persistent*.

What appears to be necessary for A's, then, is an assessment of priorities, and an ability to sort relevant from irrelevant challenge. How important is it to become aroused during a traffic jam, or to endure the internal catecholamine storm for the sake of job advancement, if the consequence could be coronary heart disease? One must make a living, you protest. Let us speak with Mr. A about that.

During the ten-day course of hospitalization, Mr. A had much time to think and review priorities. It suddenly occurred to him that if he did not have his health, his success at work was irrelevant. He began to question himself, for example, as to what he was living for, what was really important to him, how much money he really needed. After discharge he had a "heart-to-heart" talk with his rather Type A boss, who had himself been somewhat afraid after Mr. A's illness. He explained that he would like to continue working, but at a less frenetic pace, to take vacations, spend more time with his family, and in general be gentler with himself and his expectations. In thinking about it, he realized that if he were a bit lower key, he would probably get along better with his colleagues and subordinates, with resulting improved efficiency and a more pleasant working atmosphere.

Mr. A's boss was sympathetic, and approved of his intentions. Had he not, Mr. A would have had some difficult decisions to make. He could have sought other employment, which might present some difficulties in light of his health history; claimed work-related disability (with some validity) and apply for workers' compensation; or change to a less stressful occupation. he could have purchased a small piece of land in the country and lived a subsistence lifestyle, not a rare phenomenon in the area of Maine in which I once resided. Or he simply could have continued as before. The last course was the least acceptable to him.

Not all Type A's who experience infarction or new-onset angina are as amenable to change as this patient. Denial may be a prominent aspect of an A's coping methodology, and it has been hypothesized[3] that this may delay the seeking of health care by patients with coronary disease, to their detriment. Another disconcerting aspect of denial is that fatigue, anxiety, irritability, and other symptoms of overwork and excessive stress may be submerged in the drive to achieve. This tendency has been demonstrated experimentally.[8] In a purely physical survival situation, this might be lifesaving if prolonged vigilance is imperative, but it is likely to be maladaptive otherwise.

What are the barriers to altering Type A behavior, aside from "technical" considerations? Motivation is, of course, imperative, and it is hoped that this book will provide a basis for such motivation. Coronary heart disease is a preventable disease, and we have demonstrated that dimunition of risk is likely attendant to dimunition of this risk factor. It should be obvious intellectually that without health, achievement and acquisition are irrelevant. Mr. A, as do others, learn this on an emotional level as well, all too frequently after the disease is severe enough to be symptomatic, and the primary motivator is fear. Sometimes this is the fire necessary to burn through the barrier of denial.

Let us assume that our patients or clients confess to their A'ness, and no longer deny it. (This is quite common among A's, who only deny the *sequelae* of the behavior.) There are deeply ingrained societal imperatives that support and reward the type A behavior Pattern (TABP), making change difficult to initiate, even if the patient knows he or she is Type A. Competition is a watchword of life in the West from early childhood. Our heroes are fighters, athletes in competitions, glamorous, wealthy individualists who have clawed their way up out of the oblivion of the common man. Since childhood we have been graded, ranked, judged, and promoted in the basis of our ability to compete in a variety of systems, and to a variety of ends.

"A'ness" is a state of "me'ness." It is "I against the world," "I as compared with." The A's conversation is replete with self-references, and often the A evinces easily triggered hostility in the face of opposition. Meyer Freidman terms the Type A "egocentric"—that is, selfish, defined rather obviously by the preoccupation with self and self's positions or possessions in comparison with others.

In the final analysis, survival and reproduction are evolution's "bottom line." Physical survival is more readily assured in contemporary Western society than at any other time in our evolutionary history, and Type A behavior is no longer a prerequisite for attaining a reasonable level of physical comfort. Reproductive fitness does not involve physical competition as it does so frequently in the animal world. Consequently, despite our conceptions to the contrary, the Type A behavior pattern is no longer a functional genetic adaptation, and, as we have discussed, may be the opposite.

Even if one accepts the premise that being "A" may facilitate progress in the corporate and academic worlds, the cost would appear to be potentially excessive. This is the realization we must foster in our patients. The premise that "A = success" itself is questionable, and depends upon one's definition of success.

Mr. A, during the course of his retrospection, began to regret that he had been so intent on his corporate fitness that he had hurried through some of his best years and had sacrificed his present on the altar of some future executive suite he hoped to occupy. The transience of such an achievement became clear to him as he confronted the possibility of his imminent demise. His "adrenalin high" had carried him through many a board meeting, had overridden fatigue, and had allowed him to, in his perception, outcompete the more "laid back" members of the management team. He never understood how one of his colleagues had managed to attain a management position when his approach seemed so casual and "mellow," and he had inwardly despised the man for his calm and unruffled behavior under fire. Now, however, he realized that frenetic and "hyper" behavior was not necessary in order to accomplish goals. Type B's can and do succeed.

We know that outward behavior may not mirror inward arousal, and it may be that only sophisticated physiologic monitoring may detect the silent hot reactor, but I would speculate that the *symptoms* of hyperreactivity are felt by these patients, even if denied. Cold hands, rapid pulse, etc., are objective indicators probably accompanied by the same internal sensations experienced by more obvious "A's." Hot reactors, I suspect, know who they are. And it would seem that there *are* B's who are successful, and are generally less reactive individuals.

The labile hypertensive, who frequently has a genetic predisposition for this state, may, over time, insulate himself or herself from stessful circumstances by using rather blantant denial, although the data are sketchy and preliminary on this point. More effective coping tools, exercise, relaxation, and, where necessary, pharmocologic intervention may obviate this risk factor for cardiovascular disease.

In the Type A, however, and probably the silent hot reactor, as well, the underlying pathology seems to be a drive toward a goal that supersedes other considerations. The techniques discussed in the last chapter are merely attempts to diminish sympathetic output or its target organ impact—an umbrella against the storm—and are at best temporizing measures, not cures.

Allow me to advance, then, a model for Type A reform, a sort of idealized prospectus of attitudes and beliefs that incorporates the potentially useful and positive aspects of the behavior pattern and eliminates its destructive components. I will start from the perspective of an avowed, well-established "A," and chart a course around the thunderheads of inappropriate arousal.

The Type A individual lives almost exclusively in the rational mind, constantly scheming, planning, or producing, unless that mind is turned off by alcohol or drugs, a not uncommon refuge in our society. A first step for the "A" is to gain perspective on the nature of the thought processes and motivations that drive him or her. This occurred for Mr. A through his enforced inactivity during his recovery, and the vulnerability and fragility he felt as a result of his clash with a life-threatening illness. This situation encouraged him to alter his perspective on life and to reassess his priorities, prompted by the startling realization of his mortality. Barring that rather drastic method, there are other techniques for inducing contemplation in A's. Time without agenda, sitting quietly on a beach or walking in the woods, listening to and being moved by music—all promote contemplative thought and insight. One must first be willing to ask oneself certain questions: What am I living for? What are the priorities? How important is my health? Why am I in such a hurry? How much is enough? Why am I doing what I am doing? Is it injuring me? Is it my reaction to "it" or "them" that is the problem? What should I be doing for the sake of my health that I am not doing? These questions must be considered carefully, individually, and repeatedly. We as health care providers can ask our patients these questions, and insist on answers.

Such questioning often provokes significant and positive life changes without the necessity to experience a major illness. Continuing, ongoing quiet times alone are important to the type A, as to everyone. But A's particularly find it difficult to accomplish, and so setting this time aside might be undertaken initially as a discipline. If insight is forthcoming, the regime should become a natural one thereafter.

A's must also address the issue of denial. Insensitivity to physical sensations and refusal to attribute stress-related symptoms to their cause is a common "A" phenomenon. Tension headache, peptic distress, fatigue, tics, tremulousness, and irritability are all possible signals of physical overextension. Specific symptoms of arousal, such as palpitations or rapid heart rate, hyperalertness, and "butterflies," often go unrecognized or unacknowledged. This is perhaps why Mr. A was so surprised by his infarction.

I have avoided personal testimony in this book other than to allude to my own "A'ness." I wish here only to relate my intense surprise when it became apparent to me, after medical consultation, that the palpitations I was experiencing and the muscle twitch over my eye were indeed "stress related," and were a physical message from my fatigued, chronically overaroused body to my conscious mind. What was particularly fascinating was that I did not *feel* stressed; I had no subjective sense that I was overextended, fatigued, and hyperaroused, and yet, when considered logically, all of these were true. My amazement stemmed from my own subjective insulation to psychogenic overload. The extent of my denial was profound.

The corollary of this is that sensitivity to physical signals by Type A's, and others, is extremely important. This requires some degree of self-diagnostic skill, but it is not difficult to attain in that we all tend to react somewhat stereotypically in stressful circumstances, and a little insight and attentiveness will generally uncover what that constellation of symptoms is for a given individual. We can teach our patients to be their own diagnosticians of arousal, by checking their pulses, becoming aware of symptoms of vasoconstriction such as cold and clammy extremities, and monitoring their own blood pressures at home and at work. Medical consultation may be necessary if frank organic disease is in question. The absence of a sense of "anxiety" on a conscious level despite physical symptoms of stress is rather startling to one who is confronted with it—a rather common occurrence amoung patients in my practice. This awareness may provoke a reappraisal of the significance of the circumstances surrounding the arousal, defusing the importance of the situation via emotion-focused coping, or promoting an active coping strategy.

Our reforming "A" would also do well to utilize suppression to cope with certain uncontrollable events. The event is known and understood, the rules are clear, and no action is possible or advisable at the time. Consequently dwelling on the issue is likely to keep the paper tiger alive, and stimulate ongoing reactivity; for example, worrying about job problems at home or on the weekend, dwelling on fears when there is nothing that can alter circumstances at the moment, or maintaining anger when one is unable to communicate that feeling of anger to its object. Sometimes a good planning session, during which attention is directed to the problem, active coping methods are evaluated and recorded, and the issue is "internally tabled" until an appropriate time, may allow diffusion of much distress, and probably arousal.

These skills can be taught. Recognition of arousal or the potential for it in a given circumstance can be taught to initiate a cascade of thought processes. For instance, I am feeling aroused, a bit agitated and tense. I check my pulse, it is faster than usual. My hands feel cold, my mouth is dry. The circumstances surrounding this are that I am scheduled to present a report to my supervisors at work tomorrow, one of whom is hostile to me. My current thought content is how important it is that I do well so that a promotion will become more likely. I worry that no matter what I say, the supervisor will respond negatively. I cannot bear failure; job advancement is critical to me or I am worthless.

Diagnosis: arousal precipitated by a Type A relevant challenge. Therapy:

1. Assessing the true significance of the challenge—is this arousal worth the potential cost? This entails reminding myself of the risks incurred by this arousal. Certainly my job is important to me, but my health is more so. Furthermore, it is not that my job is at risk—perhaps only my self-esteem.
2. Problem-focused coping. Am I prepared for the presentation? I have rehearsed it several times, but I need two more bits of information that will not be available until just before the meeting. I have, however, made a list and I know where and when to acquire the data in the morning. I can do nothing more tonight.
3. Emotion-focused coping. There is nothing I can do about the hostile supervisor. The reality is that he does not have the final decision about my advancement in the company, and ultimately all I can do is my best and let the cards fall where they may.
4. Suppression. The meeting is not until tomorrow. It is a beautiful evening, and I am not going to ruin it by worrying. I'll put it out of my mind until morning, when I return to work.
5. Physiology. I'll go for a jog now, and in the morning before work do a short relaxation session.

Each component of this process requires work and coaxing, but nurses, therapists, or other health-care providers are in a situation to encourage such perspectives.

A's often enjoy, and seem to need, some physiologic arousal. We have alluded to the "adrenalin high," those moments of working at peak efficiency, challenged, coordinated, clear-headed, and competent. A healthful mode of incorporating this into one's life is physical arousal to physical challenge. I am not drawn to death-defying challenges, but find such sports as windsurfing, skiing, and running excellent outlets for sympathomedullary arousal. I believe it balances A's to engage in such activities, although I have no studies to quote to support this contention, but only observation of myself and others.

Work environments that are challenging and require active decision making and fast thinking are often enjoyable to A's. Here the concept of "relevant challenge" may be invoked. If the arousal is directed, is of short duration, and is not carried beyond the confines of the challenge, it may be far less damaging, and indeed utilitarian. The use of the various types of umbrellas from the last chapter may aid in limiting the extent or duration of the arousal. Most of us do not want to live boring lives, free from challenges. I commented at the beginning of this book that stress may be a positive force for growth and change. It is ascertaining the nature of relevant challenge that is the key to "A" reform, and limiting the extent of arousal afterward.

Here, again, we return to priorities: determining what matters in life and defining the nature of the goals we pursue and why we pursue them.

Viktor Frankl, the Austrian psychiatrist and author of *Man's Search for Meaning*, a chronicle of the Nazi holocaust and of his experiences in a concentration camp, discovered that those who survived had one factor in common: an overwhelming reason to do so—for someone or something else. For him it was the hope of seeing his family again, and the need to communicate his observations on this atrocity to the world. For others it might be the life of a family member or members, or perhaps work left undone —whatever they considered a totally compelling reason to endure, a reason for living. This brilliant man created an entire mode of psychotherapy—logotherapy—on the basis of his observations.

Most physicians who deal with the critically ill, including myself, have noticed that those who have a strong desire to survive tend to do so, or at least to cling more tenaciously to life, than those who have given up.

What this has to do with Type A reform is that the Type A pattern is fundamentally acquisitive, and "A" goals are often directed in that way. Purpose in life other than acquisition is, in my estimation, a stronger motivator for survival, as Mr. A may have discovered. Indeed, much of his insight seemed to have stemmed from that realization. If survival becomes important to an individual because that individual has something to live for, whether family, cause, or creation, then classic Type A behavior, with its aggressiveness, hostility, time urgency, and competitiveness, is antisurvival. Recall, again, how the presence of the pattern alone more than doubles the risk of coronary disease. The silent hot reactor might think of himself or herself in these terms, as well.

Physician and nonphysician health-care providers can be of tremendous help to the cardiovascular hot reactor. We can assist in making the diagnosis by aiding self-assessment and rendering our own objective opinions about the individual's behavior and risks for arousal. We can educate the patient about the consequences of an aroused physiologic state evoked by psychological challenge. We can explore the nature of those challenges and their potency. We can teach awareness of physical symptoms and their meaning. We can teach coping methods, ways of diffusing the significance of events, and tools to take the sting out of sympathomedullary arousal. And we can add a dimension of healing to the patient afflicted with coronary disease that transcends physical considerations and may promote some rather profound life-style changes that will lead to a happier, healthier existence.

It is clear that there are no easy methods here, no crystal-clear answers, no untarnished absolute truths. There are, however, patterns, suggestions, and consistencies that lead us to believe that certain ways of reacting to the environment are unhealthful at the least and potentially fatal at worst, but are amenable to change. Such change is not easy or rapid, but would appear to have great value, not only in the prophylaxis of disease, but in the improvement of the quality of life as well.

Life is too short to hurry through it.

REFERENCES

1. Folkman, S. Personal control and stress and coping processes: A theoretical analysis. *J Pers Soc Psychol*, 46:839–852, 1984.
2. Rotter, J. B. Some problems and misconceptions related to the construct of internal versus external control of reinforcement. *J Consult Clin Psychol*, 43:56–67, 1875.
3. Pittner, M. S., and Houston, K. B. Response to stress, cognitive coping strategies, and the Type A behavior pattern. *J Pers Soc Psychol*, 39:147–157, 1980.
4. Rothbaum, F., Weisz, J. R., and Snyder, S. S. Changing the world and changing the self: A two process model of perceived control. *J Pers Soc Psychol*, 42:5–37, 1982.
5. Light, K. C. Cardiovascular responses to active effortful coping: Implications for the role of stress in hypertension development. *Psychophysiology*, 18:216–225, 1981.
6. Manuck, S. B., Harvey, A. E., et al. Effects of active coping on blood pressure responses to threat of aversive stimulation. *Psychophysiology*, 15:544–549, 1978.
7. Matthews, K. A. Psychological peerspectives on the Type A behavior pattern. *Psychol Bull*, 91:293–323, 1983.
8. Carver, C. S., Coleman, A. E., and Glass, D. C. The coronoary-prone behavior and suppression of fatigue on a treadmill test. *J Pers Soc Psychol*, 33:460–466, 1976.

GLOSSARY

Alpha-receptors: Those receptors of the sympathetic nervous system that, when stimulated, cause constriction of most arteries.
Angina pectoris: The pain syndrome caused by inadequate blood supply to the heart.
Arrhythmia: An abnormal heart rythym.
Atherosclerosis: The process of progressive occlusion of the arteries of the body by plaques of cholesterol, calcium, scar tissue, and blood clots.
Autonomic nervous system: The division of the nervous system responsible for unconscious or "involuntary" functions, such as distribution of blood, organ function, and various metabolic activities. Composed of sympathetic and parasympathetic components.
Beta-blocker: A medication that blocks the beta-receptors of the sympathetic nervous system in such a way that they, when stimulated by epinephrine or nerepinephrine, fail to respond.
Beta-receptors: Those receptors of the sympathetic nervous system that, when stimulated, increase the force and speed of the heart, open the airways, mobilize fuel, and dilate blood vessels supplying skeletal muscles.
Biofeedback: A technique for learning to control "involuntary" body functions such as heart rate or blood pressure.
Cardiac catheterization: The process of threading a catheter through an artery of the body to the heart, where dye is injected into the coronary arteries and x-rays taken to determine the extent of blockage of those arteries by atherosclerosis. Also known as coronary angiography.

GLOSSARY

Catecholamines: Generic term for the effectors of the sympathetic nervous system, primarily epinephrine and norepinephrine.

Coping: Behavioral or cognitive methods of dealing with stressful stimuli.

Coronary heart disease (coronary artery disease): Atherosclerosis of the coronary arteries, the feeder arteries of the heart muscle.

Diuretic: A medication that increases salt and water loss by the kidney, diminishing vascular volume, and hence blood pressure.

Epinephrine: A hormone released by the adrenal medulla that stimulates a "fight-or-flight" stress response, essentially complementing sympathetic nervous activation. Also known as adrenaline.

Homeostasis: The maintenance of a constant internal environment.

Hormone: A chemical substance released by a gland into the blood stream that stimulates cells or organs to respond in a specific fashion.

Hyperkinetic: A physiologic stress response characterized primarily by an increase in heart rate and force of contraction. Mediated primarily by beta-receptors.

Hypertension, essential: A disease of unknown cause characterized by fixed blood pressure elevation.

Hypertension, labile: A condition in which blood pressure readings fluctuate from normal to elevated from day to day. A family history of essential hypertension is often present. Felt to be a prodromal stage of the latter.

Hypertonic: A physiologic stress response characterized primarily by constriction of blood vessels. Mediated primarily by alpha-receptors.

Ischemia: Deficient oxygen supply to a tissue or organ.

Jenkins Activity Survey: A self-administered questionnaire utilized for diagnosing and quantitating the Type A behavior pattern. Standardized primarily for urban middle-class males.

Myocardial infarction: Death of heart muscle resulting from interruption of blood flow, usually as a result of coronary heart disease. Also known as a heart attack.

Myocardium: Heart muscle.

Neurotransmitter: A substance released at the junction between nerve and nerve or nerve and organ that stimulates a response from the receiving structure.

Norepinephrine: A neurotransmitter released by nerves of the sym-

pathetic nervous system that stimulates the "fight-or-flight" stress response.
Parasympathetic nervous system: The counterpoint of the sympathetic nervous system, responsible for vegetative functions such as digestion. When stimulated results in salivation, increased bowel activity, and decreased heart rate, among many other actions.
Premature ventricular contraction: An extra heart beat, originating in the ventricle instead of the atrium, often associated with electrical irritability of the heart. Also known as extrasystole.
Renin: A hormone released by the kidney, generally in response to lowered blood pressure, but also in response to stress in some individuals, that promotes retention of salt and water by the kidney and hence raises the blood pressure.
Structured interview: A standardized interview designed to evoke components of the Type A behavior pattern for diagnostic purposes. Audio or video recordings are often employed for later analysis. Generally considered the "gold standard" for diagnosis of this pattern.
S-T depression: An electrocardiographic finding that may indicate myocardial ischemia.
Sympathetic nervous system: A division of the autonomic nervous system responsible for activating the organism physically to respond to a stressful situation.
Sympathomedullary arousal: Activation of the sympathetic nervous system and release of epinephrine from the adrenal medulla, generally in response to stress.
Ventricular fibrillation: An arrythmia characterized by chaotic electrical impulses such that the heart does not beat effectively. If not immediately treated, it is invariably fatal, and is the most common cause of sudden death.

Name Index

Adams, D. F., 71, 73, 74
Adler, R. H., 134
Agras, W. S., 149, 151
Alexander, F., 78
Allen, M. T., 53, 54, 69, 80
Andrews, G., 141
Angulo, J., 54
Appels, A., 31
Arabian, J. M., 55, 56
Archibald, D. G., 89
Aslan, S., 53, 56

Bajusz, E., 94
Bali, L. R., 150
Barefoot, J. C., 38
Barker, G. F., 94
Beane, W. E., 39
Becker, M. A., 39
Bengtsson, C., 31
Benson, H., 148
Berman, R., 93
Black, G. M., 127
Black, W. C., 94
Blakelock, E. H., 77, 78
Block, P., 36
Bloom, L. J., 121
Blumenthal, J. A., 28, 30, 35, 51, 127, 143, 144
Boyer, J. L., 141
Bradis, V. A., 102
Brammell, H. L., 136, 143, 144
Brand, R. J., 30, 32, 91
Braunwald, E., 72

Brod, J., 71, 73
Bruhn, J. G., 103
Brunner, D., 138
Brunson, B., 30
Brunson, J. G., 93
Bruell, J. C., 57, 81, 97
Burchell, H. B., 94
Burgess, M., 77, 79
Burnett, J., 93
Butensky, A., 54, 59
Byers, S. O., 47

Cade, R., 142
Cahen, R., 135
Callahan, K. S., 131
Campbell, W. B., 131
Cannon, A., 93
Cannon, W. B., 24, 102
Carruthers, M., 132, 134, 150
Case, D. B., 149
Case, N. B., 123
Case, R. B., 123
Chandler, B., 103
Chaplin, J. P., 94
Chave, S. P. W., 138
Chesney, A. P., 77, 78
Chesney, M. A., 27, 28, 32
Chiang, B. N., 103
Choquette, G., 142
Clarkson, T. B., 95
Clough, D., 93
Cochrane, R., 79
Cohen, J. B., 33, 34

175

NAME INDEX

Corbalan, R., 103
Corse, C. D., 57
Cottier, C., 150, 152
Cox, J. P., 146
Craft, S., 49, 52, 128
Cuomo, S., 92

Dahlstrom, W. G., 38
D'Alonzo, C. A., 103
Davia, J. E., 131, 134, 135
Davis, C. M., 48
Davis, J. W., 89
Deanfield, J. E., 98
De Caprio, L., 92
Dembrowski, T. M., 30, 38, 49, 52, 56, 128
De Mendonca, M., 73
de Servi, S., 97, 98
DeSilva, R. A., 103
de Suto-Nagy, G. I., 93
Devereux, R. B., 120
Dimsdalae, J. E., 36, 90, 132
Drury, A., 90
Dunbar, H. F., 26
Duncan, C. H., 102
Durel, L. A., 131, 134, 135
Dyck, D. G., 128

Eaker, E. D., 33, 34
Eich, R. H., 72
Eliasson, K., 69, 71, 81
Eliot, R. S., 81, 97
Elliot, D. L., 143
Elmadjian, F., 46, 57, 79
Engel, B. T., 149
Engel, G. L., 99, 101, 105
Erfurt, J. C., 77, 78
Esler, M., 75, 77
Evens, J. F., 146

Fabrega, H., 91, 92, 93
Falchone, C., 97, 98
Falkner, B., 69, 71, 80
Fani, K., 89
Faralli, V., 54, 59
Federman, D., 64
Feinleib, M., 32, 33, 34
Ferguson, R. J., 142
Ferrans, V. J., 93, 94
Fisher, R., 102

Fleming, J., 135
Folkman, S., 158
Folkow, B., 76
Folsom, A. R., 113
Francois, B., 135
Frank, K., 35, 37
Frankel, B. L., 149
Fredrikson, M., 70, 71
Friedman, G. D., 33, 34
Friedman, M., 29, 30, 32, 46, 47, 121
Friedrich, G., 131, 134, 135
Frumkin, K., 149
Furedy, J. J., 51

Gaarder, K. R., 149
Gambaro, S., 77, 79
Ganelina, I. E., 31
Garland, F. N., 51
Gastorf, J. W., 50
Gemzell, C. A., 46
Gentry, W. D., 77, 78
Gershengorn, K., 89
Gibbons, D., 98
Gifford, R. W., 113, 117
Gill, J. J., 121
Gillum, R. F., 113
Glass, D., 38
Gold, K. J., 49, 52, 128
Goldband, S., 49
Goldberg, L., 143
Goldring, D., 141
Goldstein, D., 71
Gordon, D. J., 143
Grascow, M. S., 149
Gravejat, M. J., 135
Green, H. J., 135
Groen, 71, 73, 76, 81

Hackett, T., 36
Haft, J. I., 89, 94, 95
Hagberg, J. M., 141
Hallstrom, T., 31
Hamer, J., 135
Hancock, W., 27
Handforth, C. P., 94
Haney, T., 37
Harburg, E., 77, 78
Harshfield, G. A., 120
Hartley, H., 132

NAME INDEX

Hartley, L. H., 90, 97
Hartwell, A., 93
Harvey, A. E., 160
Harvey, W. P., 101
Hastrup, J. L., 69, 80
Hauenstein, L., 77, 78
Haynes, S. G., 33, 34
Heady, J. A., 137
Heidbreder, E., 135
Heidland, A., 135
Heimreich, R. L., 39
Heiss, G., 142
Heller, S., 35, 37, 123
Herd, A. J., 90
Herlitz, J., 131
Herman, S., 127
Heslegrave, R. L., 51
Hiatt, W. R., 136
Hibbs, R. G., 93, 94
Highman, B., 94
Hjalmarson, A., 131
Hjemdahl, P., 69, 71, 81
Hjermann, I., 123
Hofer, M. A., 105
Hokanson, J. E., 77, 79
Holland, O. B., 116
Hollenberg, N. K., 71, 73, 74
Holme, I., 123
Hope, J. M., 46, 57, 79
Horne, M., 149, 151
Horowitz, D., 149
Houston, B. K., 50, 63, 69
Houston, K., 30
Houston, K. B., 159
Hovig, T., 89
Hueper, W. C., 95
Hugenholtz, P., 92
Hughson, R. L., 135
Hull, E. M., 144
Hunninghake, D., 143
Hutter, A. M., 36
Hyde, R. T., 138, 139

Jamieson, J. L., 146
Janisse, M. P., 128
Jenkins, C. D., 29, 30, 32, 33, 34
Johansson, B. W., 116
Johansson, G., 94
Johnson, A. R., 131
Johnson, H. H., 39
Johnson, N. J., 142
Jonsson, L., 94
Jorgensen, L., 89
Jorgensen, R., 63, 69
Julius, S., 150, 152

Kahn, J. P., 55
Kalis, B., 76
Kannel, W. B., 33, 34
Kaplan, J. R., 95
Kaplan, N. M., 113
Kappeli, L., 134
Karvonen, M. J., 139
Kasch, F. W., 141
Keane, T. M., 71
Kearney, H., 121
Keller, S., 145, 146
Keys, A., 139
King, W. M., 93
Kittel, F., 30
Klatsky, A. L., 33, 34
Kline, I. K., 94
Kong, Y., 28, 30, 35
Konstantinos, M., 142
Kornfeld, D., 35, 37, 55
Kornitzer, M., 30
Kraevsky, Y. M., 31
Krantz, D. S., 38, 52, 55, 56, 131, 134, 135
Kranz, P. D., 89
Kraus, W. E., 136
Krifcher, E., 71
Krotkiewski, M., 142
Kuhnert, L., 116
Kuller, L., 102

Laman, C., 36
Lamson, E. T., 46, 57, 79
Lane, J. D., 51, 52, 82
Lang, C. M., 95
Lawler, J. E., 71, 94, 103
Lawler, K. A., 53, 54, 69, 80
Lee, K., 37
Lee, K. T., 103
Lee, W. M., 103
Leon, A. S., 137, 138, 139, 146, 147
Levine, S. A., 101
Lewis, H. D., Jr., 89

177

NAME INDEX

Lie, J. T., 103
Light, K. C., 69, 73, 80, 160
Lilienfield, A., 102
Lobitz, C. W., 143, 144
Lorimer, A. R., 71, 75
Lown, B., 103
Luepker, R. V., 113
Lundberg, U., 54
Lund-Johnson, P., 136
Lushene, R., 49, 56
Lyle, A. M., 103

MacDougall, J. M., 30, 38, 49, 52, 56, 128
MacFarlane, B. J., 135
MacMahon, S. W., 141
Malcolm, A. T., 128
Malek, I., 131
Maling, H. M., 94
Manelis, G., 138
Manuck, S. B., 49, 51, 52, 57, 95, 128, 160
Marmot, M. G., 150, 152
Mars, D., 142
Marsh, R. C., 136
Marzetta, B. R., 148
Matta, R. J., 103
Matthews, K., 30, 38, 39, 54, 160
McCloud, A. A., 136
McKelvain, R., 36
Mehlman, B., 93
Melville, D., 69, 70, 71, 72, 80
Menninger, K. A., 26
Menninger, W. C., 26
Mills, D. C. B., 96
Mitchell, B., 92, 93
Modan, M., 138
Mohr, C., 102
Morris, J. N., 137, 138
Moss, A. J., 93, 94
Moss, L., 90
Moss, S., 138
Moutsos, S. E., 71

Nahas, G. G., 93
Nathan, R. J., 149
Neftel, K. A., 134
Nelson, L., 53, 56
Nestel, P. J., 71

Neus, H., 131, 134, 135
Nixon, J. V., 116
North, W. R. S., 149

Obrist, P. A., 69, 80
Osler, W., 26
Ovcharchyn, C. A., 39

Paffenberger, R. S., 138, 139
Pagel, G., 135
Paredes, A., 103
Patel, C., 149, 150, 152
Patel, D. J., 149
Pell, S., 103
Perlman, L. V., 103
Peronnet, F., 146
Petzel, T. P., 39
Pickering, T. G., 120
Pittner, M. S., 30, 50, 159
Pollack, A. A., 149
Pratt, C. M., 136
Prout, M. F., 149

Raab, W., 93, 94
Rabin, A. I., 77, 79
Raffle, P. A. B., 137
Raftery, E. B., 69, 70
Ram, sC. V. S., 117
Ray, W. J., 48
Reich, P., 101
Reid, J., 116
Reiland, S., 142
Reiser, M. F., 72, 76
Remington, R., 32, 63, 69
Rixse, A., 53
Robb, J. A., 96
Roberts, G. K., 96
Roeper, P. J., 77, 78
Rosenman, R., 27, 28, 29, 30, 32, 38, 91
Roskies, E., 120, 121
Rosner, B. A., 148
Ross, A., 69, 71, 72, 80
Rothbaum, F., 159
Rotter, J. B., 158
Rowsell, H. C., 89
Rubenstein, E., 64, 76
Ruskin, J., 132
Ryan, T. J., 34

NAME INDEX

Sable, D. L., 136
St. George, S., 46
Sapira, J. D., 71, 76
Schenk, E. A., 93, 94
Scherwitz, L., 36
Schiffer, F., 97
Schmieder, R., 131, 134, 135
Schonfeld, G., 142
Schwaratz, P. J., 51
Schwartz, S. G., 146
Seer, P., 149
Seraganian, P., 145
Shapiro, A., 71, 92, 93
Shapiro, K., 150, 152
Shields, J. L., 128
Shinebourne, E., 135
Sigler, L. H., 93
Sime, W. E., 57, 97
Simons, H., 92
Simonson, E., 93
Singer, M., 72, 76
Sinyor, D., 146
Sjostrom, L., 142
Skinner, J. E., 103
Snyder, S. S., 159
Somerville, W., 98, 132, 134
Sontag, S., 4, 5
Spain, D. M., 102
Specchia, G., 97, 98
Spevack, M., 120, 121
Squires, W. G., 136
Steptoe, A., 69, 71, 72, 80
Stern, R. M., 48
Stevenson, I. P., 102
Stewart, I. M. G., 26
Stoll, S., 143, 144
Struthers, A., 116
Suinn, R. M., 121
Sullivan, P., 71, 78
Suls, J., 39
Surkis, A., 120, 121
Svensson, J. C., 71, 73
Syme, S. L., 33, 34

Szakacs, J. E., 93

Taggart, P., 98, 132, 134
Taylor, C. B., 149, 151
Terry, D. J., 150, 152
Theorell, T., 71, 73
Thompson, P. L., 103
Thoreson, C. E., 121
Tibbin, G., 31
Titus, J. L., 94

Ury, H. K., 33, 34

Van Dusch, T., 26
Van Egeren, L. F., 91, 92, 93
Van Vliet, P. D., 94
Velve Byre, K., 123
Verrier, R., 103
Von Euler, U. S., 46, 79

Waldron, I., 53
Walford, R., 2
Waters, I. L., 93
Weber, M. A., 149
Weiner, H., 72, 76
Weiss, T., 51
Weisz, J. R., 159
Welton, D. E., 136
White, A. D., 52
Whitesmith, R., 116
Williams, G. H., 71, 73, 74
Williams, R., 28, 30, 35, 37
Williams, R. B., 38, 82, 143, 144
Williams, R. S., 136, 143, 144
Wing, A. L., 138, 139
Witztum, J., 142, 143
Wolf, S., 102, 103, 104
Wrzesniewski, K., 30

Young, S. H., 144

Ziegler, M. G., 144
Zyzanski, S., 30, 32, 34, 53

Subject Index

Activity, *see* Exercise
Activity Survey, 172
   Type A behavior pattern and, 29, 30
Acute stress, 11-12
Adaptability
   definition of, 8
   perception of stressor and, 10-11
Adaptation
   as "cure" for stress, 11
   definition of, 8
   homeostasis and, 8-9
Adrenal gland, 15
Adrenalin, *see* Epinephrine
Adrenergic nervous system, *see* Sympathetic nervous system
Aerobic fitness training, 143-147, *see also* Exercise
Afterload, 120
Age, Type A behavior pattern and, 53-54
Alpha-blockers, 136-137
Alpha-receptors, 19-21
   definition of, 171
Anger, *see also* Hostility
   inhibition of, hypertension and, 77-79
Angina pectoris, 30-31, *see also* Coronary heart disease
   definition of, 171
Angiogram, 31, 34-37

Anxiety, beta-blockers and, 134
Appraisal, 158
Arousal, *see* Sympathomedullary arousal
Arrhythmia, 98-99, 100
   blood pressure control efficacy and, 116
   definition of, 171
   sudden death and, 102-103
Arteriogram, 31, 34-37
Atherosclerosis, 88-89, *see also* Coronary heart disease
   cholesterol and, 90
   definition of, 171
   hyperreactivity and, 95-96
   risk of, reduction of, *see* Interventions
Autonomic nervous system, definition of, 171

Behavioral intervention, 120-124, 164-169
   passive, 147-151
Beta-blockers, 129-136
   anxiety and, 134
   definition of, 171
   exercise and, 135
   hypertension and, 130, 134-135
   previous myocardial infarction and, 130-131
   Type A behavior pattern and, 131-135

181

SUBJECT INDEX

Beta-receptors, 21
  definition of, 171
  types of, 129
Biofeedback, 148, 149-151
  definition of, 171
Blood clotting, atherosclerotic lesions and, 89
Blood pressure, see also Hypertension
  cardiovascular reactivity patterns and, 81, 82
  fall in, fight-o-flight phenomenon and, 105
  Type A behavior and, 49, 57
Blood pressure control
  beta-blockers in, 130 see also Beta-blockers
  diuretics in, 137
  efficacy of, 112-120
    arrhythmias and, 116
    cardiac hypertrophy and, 120
    HDFP and, 114-119
    mild hypertensives and, 113, 118-119
    MRFIT and, 115-119
    target organ damage and, 118
  exercise in, 140-142
  nonpharmacologic approach to, passive, 148-151
Blood vessel walls, catecholamine effects on, 95-96
Body systems, requirements of, 7
Body temperature, homeostasis of, 7-8
Borderline hypertensives, see Prehypertensives
Brain, sympathomedullary arousal and, 21-22

Cardiac arrhythmia, see Arrhythmia
Cardiac catheterization, definition of, 171
Cardiac hypertrophy, 120
Cardiac rehabilitation exercise, 147

Cardioselective drugs, 129, see also Beta-blockers
Cardiovascular disease, see Coronary heart disease
Cardiovascular reactivity, see also Hyperreactivity
  exercise and, 144-147
  patterns of, 81, 82
Catecholamines, 87 see also Sympathomedullary arousal; specific catecholamine
  blood vessel walls and, 95-96
  cardiac damage caused by, 91-94
  definition of, 172
  exercise and, 145
  known coronary heart disease anad, 97-99
  rhythm disorders and, 98-99, 103
  sudden death and, 103, 104
  Type A behavior pattern and, 46-47
Catecholamine storm, 94
Catheterization, cardiac, 171
Children, Type A behavior in, 54
Cholesterol level
  episodic elevations of, 90-91
  exercise and, 142-143
  Type A behavior pattern and, 35
Chronic stress
  intermittent, 12
  persistent, 12-13
Clotting, atherosclerotic lesions and, 89
Cognitive intervention, 120-124
Conservation withdrawal, 104-105
Control, secondary, 159-160
Coping, 158-164
  controllability and, 158, 161
  definition of, 158, 172
  denial in, 159, 162-163, 165-166
  emotion-focused, 159
  problem-focused, 159
  secondary control in, 159-160
  strategies for, reactivity

SUBJECT INDEX

correlates of, 160-164
suppression in, 159
Coronaray angiogram, 31, 34-37
Coronary heart disease, 87-106
   catecholamines and, 91-96
      known disease and, 97-99
   cholesterol and, 90-91
   definition of, 172
   diagnosis of, 30-31
   palpitations in, 99
   pathogenesis of, 64-66
   platelets and, 89
   populations at risk for, 111-112
   risk of, reduction of, 111-124, *see also* Interventions
   sudden death and, 99-105
      psychological profile and, 103-104
   Type A behavior and, 25-40, *see also* Type A behavior pattern
Counseling Type A intervention with, 122-123

Death, sudden, 99-105
   during exercise, 146-147
   psychological profile and, 103-104
Denial, 159, 162-163, 165-166
Disease, stress-related, 2, 4-5, 44-45, *see also specific disease*
Diuretics, 137
   beta-blockers versus, 131
   definition of, 172
Drugs, 129-137, *see also* Medications; *specific type*

Eggocentrism, 163
Electrocardiogram
   blood pressure control efficacy and, 116
   in cardiac damage assessment, catecholamine toxicity and, 91-93
   in coronary heart disease diagnosis, 31
Electrophysiologic monitoring, of

hyperreactivity, Type A behavior pattern and, 48-49
Emotion-focused coping, 159
Energy, 18
Environment, adaptation to, 8-9
Epinephrine, 15, 19, 20, *see also* Catecholamines
   cardiac damage caused by, 93-94
   definition of, 172
Essential hypertension, 67, 172, *see also* Hypertension
Estivation, 104-105
Exercise, 137-147
   beta-blockers and, 135
   catecholamines and, 145
   cholesterol and, 142-143
   hypertension and, 140-142
   sudden death during, 146-147
   Type A behavior pattern and, 143-145
Exercise-tolerance test, 91, 147
Extrasystole, 99, 100, *see also* Arrhythmia
   sudden death and, 102-103

Fainting, conservation withdrawal and, 105
Family history, essential hypertension and, 69
Feedback loop, 22-23, 24
Fight-or-flight phenomenon, 15, 66, *see also* Physiology of stress response; Sympathomedullary arousal
   beta-blockers and, 135, *see also* Beta-blockers
   counterpoint of, 104-105
   hormone release and, 18
Fitness training, 143-147, *see also* Exercise
Framingham study, 32-33

Gender, Type A behavior and, 52-54

HDFP (Hypertension Detection and Followup Program), 114-119

SUBJECT INDEX

HDL (high-density lipoprotein), exercise and, 142-143
Heart disease, see also Coronary heart disease
  hypertensive, 120
Heart rate, Type A behavior and, 49
Hibernation, 104-105
High-density lipoprotein (HDL), exercise and, 142-143
Homeostasis, 7-10
  definition of, 172
  feedback loop and, 22-23, 24
Hormone(s)
  definition of, 172
  neurotransmitter versus, 15-17
  stress response and, 18
Ho scale, 37-38
Hostility, see also Type A behavior pattern
  coronary heart disease and, 37-38
  hyperreactivity and, challenge and, 52
  suppression of, hypertension and, 77-79
Hyperkinetic reactivity, 81, 82, 172
  blood pressure and, 81-83
Hyperreactivity, see also Sympathomedullary arousal; Type A behavior pattern
  atherosclerosis and, 95-96
  cardiovascular, 46
  hostility and, 52
  interventions in, see Interventions
  Type A, prehypertensive versus, 81
Hypertension, 67-83, see also Blood pressure
  anger inhibition and, 77-79
  control of, see Blood pressure control
  definition of, 67-68
  elements of, 68
  essential of, 172
  hyporeactivity in, 76-77
  labile, 172, see also Prehypertensives
  model of, 79-80
  progression of, stages in, 72
  salt and water retention in, 73-74
  sympathomedullary arousal and, 68, 70-71
  patterns of, 73
Hypertension Detection and Followup Program (HDFP), 114-119 Hypertensive heart disease, 120
Hypertonic reactivity, 81, 82, 172
Hyporeactivity, hypertension and, 76-77

Illness, stress-related, 2, 4-5, 44-45, see also specific illness
Intermittent stress, chronic, 12
Interventions, 111-124, 127-152, see also specific type
  aims of, 112
  behavioral, 120-124, 164-169
  passive, 147-151
  cognitive, 120-124
  efficacy of, 112-120
  exercise, 137-147
  pharmacologic, 129-137, see also Medications
Ischemia, definition of, 172

Jenkins Activity Survey, 172
  Type A behavior pattern and, 29, 30

Kidney, renin release by, blood pressure and, 68

Labile hypertension, see also Prehypertensives
  definition of, 172
LDL (low-density lipoprotein), exercise and, 143
Leisure exercise, see also Exercise
  sedentary life-style versus, 138

SUBJECT INDEX

Lipoproteins, *see also* Cholesterol level
  exercise and, 142-143
Low-density lipoprotein (LDL), exercise and, 143

Medications, 129-137
  alpha-blockers, 136-137
  beta-blockers, 129-136, *see also* Beta-blockers
  diuretic, 137
  hypertension treatment with, 130
Meditation, 148, 149
Mental stress
  coronary heart disease and, 98
  extrasystole and, 102-103
Mixed reactivity, 81
Mortality, *see* Death
Multiple Risk Factor Intervention Trial (MRFIT), 115-119
Muscle-relaxation techniques, 148-151
Myocardial infarction, *see also* Coronary heart disease
  definition of, 172
Myocardium, definition of, 172

Nervous system
  autonomic, 171
  parasympathetic, 18, 19, 173
  sympathetic, 18, 19-21, 173, *see also* Sympathetic nervous system
Neurotransmitter(s)
  definition of, 172
  hormone versus, 15-17
Norepinephrine, 15, 19, 20, *see also* Catecholamines
  definition of, 172-173

Occupational exercise, *see also* Exercise
  sedentary work versus, 137-138
Oxygen, 18-19

Palpitations, 99, 100
  sudden death and, 102-103

Parasympathetic nervous system, 18, 19
  conservation withdrawal and, 104-105
  definition of, 173
Passive behavioral interventions, 147-151
Perceptual alterations, 112
Persistent stress, chronic, 12-13
Pharmacologic interventions, 129-137, *see also* Medications; *specific type of medication*
Pheochromocytoma, 93-94
Physical exercise, *see* Exercise
Physical outlets, 112
Physiologic hyperresponsiveness, *see* Hyperreactivity; Type A behavior pattern
Physiology of stress response, 15-24
  adrenal gland in, 15
  alpha-receptors in, 19-21
  beta-receptors in, 21
  brain in, 21-22
  feedback loop in, 22-23, 24
  fight-or-flight phenomenon and, 15
  hormones in, 15-18
  oxygen in, 18-19
  parasympathetic nervous system in, 19
  prioritization in, 23
  sympathetic nervous system in, 19-21
  Type A behavior and, 56, *see also* Type A behavior pattern
  vascular system in, 18
Platelets
  beta-blockers and, 131
  in coronary heart disease, 64, 89
Potassium level, diuretics and, 137
Prehypertensives, 68-69, *see also* Hypertension
  hyperkinetic reactivity in, 81-83

185

SUBJECT INDEX

sympathomedullary arousal and, 70-71
Type A's versus, 80
vascular resistance in, 73
Premature contraction, 99, 100, 173, *see also* Arrhythmia
sudden death and, 102-103
Primary appraisal, 158
Priorities, assessment of, 161
Prioritization, in physiology of stress response, 23
Problem-focused coping, 159
Progressive relaxation, 148-151
Propranolol, Type A behavior pattern and, 131-132
Psychogenic stress
coronary heart disease and, 98
extrasystole and, 102-103
Psychological profile, sudden death and, 103-104

Reactivity, *see also* Hyperreactivity; Hyporeactivity; Type A behavior pattern
cardiovascular
exercise and, 144-147
patterns of, 81, 82
Relaxation techniques, 148-151
Renin
blood pressure and, 68
definition of, 173
Rhythm disorders, 100
blood pressure control efficacy and, 116
catecholamines and, 98-99, 103
sudden death and, 102-103
Rosenman and Friedman Structured Interview, 173
Type A behavior pattern and, 30

Salt retention, 73-74
Science, imprecision of, 3-5
Secondary control, 159-160
Sedentary state, exercise versus, 137-138, *see also* Exercise

Self, preoccupation with, 163
Self-ratings, of Type A characteristics, 127-129
Sex differences, Type A behavior and, 52-54
Sham death, 104-105
Silent hot reactors, *see also* Reactivity
self-assessment of, 128
"Sisyphus reaction," 104
Society, stress in, 1-2
Stress
acute, 11-12
chronic
intermittent, 12
persistent, 12-13
definition of, 10
relativity of, 10-11
Stress exercise, 91, 147
Stressor(s)
active versus passive, 70
controllability of, 158
definition of, 9-10
Stressor-stress response concept, 44-51
catecholamines and, Type A behavior pattern and, 46-47
electrophysiologic monitoring of, 48-49
perceived versus actual challenge and, 49-50
sympathomedullary arousal in, Type A behavior pattern and, 44-46
task incentive and, 50-51
threatening circumstances and, 50
Type A versus Type B individuals and, 47-48, 50-51
Stress response, *see also* Stressor-stress response concept; Sympathomedullary arousal
definition of, 10
physiology of, 15-24, *see also* Physiology of stress response
Structured Interview, 173

186

SUBJECT INDEX

Type A behavior pattern and, 30
ST-segment depression, 91-93, 173
Success, definition of, 163
Sudden death, 99-105
  during exercise, 146-147
  psychological profile and, 103-104
Suppression, 159
Sympathetic blockade, 112, *see also* Alpha-blockers; Beta-blockers
Sympathetic nervous system, 18, 19
  definition of, 173
  feedback loop and, 23, 24
  receptors in, 19-21
Sympathomedullary arousal, 21, 66, *see also* Catecholamines; Fight-or-flight phenomenon; Hyperreactivity
  blockade of, *see* Sympathetic blockade
  definition of, 173
  healthful outlets for, 168
  hypertension and, 68, *see also* Hypertension
  toxicity of, 88, *see also* Coronary heart disease
  Type A behavior pattern and, 44-46, *see also* Type A behavior pattern

TABP, *see* Type A behavior pattern
Task incentive, cardiovascular reactivity and, 50-51
Therapy, *see* Interventions; *specific type*
Thrombosis, platelets and, 89
Tranquilization, 112
Transcendental meditation, 148
Treadmill test, 91, 147
Treatment, *see* Interventions; *specific type*
Type A behavior pattern (TABP)
  appraisal and, 158
  beta-blockers and, 131-135
  blood pressure and, 57
  in children, 54
  coping with, 158-164, *see also* Coping
  coronary heart disease and, 25-40
    angiographic studies of, 34-37
    cardiovascular hyperreactivity and, 55-58
    contradictory researach on, 36-37
    hostility and, 37-38
    incidence studies of, 32
    other risk factors compared with, 35
    prevalence studies of, 31-32
    prospective studies of, 32-33
    severity of, 34-35
    sex differences in, 52-54
    specific Type A components and, 51-52
    stressor-stress response concept and, 44-51, *see also* Stressor-stress response concept
  description of, 27-28
  developmental progress of, 59
  diagnosis of, 29-30
  exercise and, 143-145
  hypertension and, 67-83, *see also* Hypertension
  interventions in, 120-124, *see also* Interventions
  passive, 147-151
  model for reform of, 164-169
  positive aspects of, 39
  prehypertensive behavior versus, 80
  reasons for, 63
  self-recognition of, 127-129
Type B behavior pattern, 28
  Type A versus, 47-48, 50-51

SUBJECT INDEX

Vascular resistance, 73
Vascular system, 18
  catecholamines and, 95-96
  prehypertensives and, 73
Ventricular fibrillation, 102, 103,
  see also Premature
    contraction
  definition of, 173
Ventricular hypertrophy, 120
Voodoo death, 102

Water pills, see Diuretics
Water retention, 73-74
Wear-and-tear hypothesis, 67
Western Collaborative Group
    Study (WCGS), 32
Work-related activity, sedentary
    work versus, 137-138, see
    also Exercise